THE MOST SERIOUS HEALTH PROBLEM IN THE UNITED STATES

is heart disease. It is now responsible for 50 percent of all deaths, with over a million Americans dying each year, and approximately 25,000 children born annually with abnormal hearts.

In clear language for the laymen to understand—and the physician to use—Dr. Shute describes diagnostic symptoms and the sometimes astonishing results of treatment with vitamin E. He also describes other conditions in which vitamin E has been helpful—diabetes, high blood pressure, severe burns, miscarriages, and more. He discusses *preventive* care, perhaps most important of all.

Here is a basic book for anyone interested in his own health and the health of his children!

VITAMIN E
FOR AILING AND HEALTHY HEARTS

by

WILFRID E. SHUTE, B.A., M.D.

with

HARALD J. TAUB

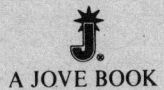

A JOVE BOOK

VITAMIN E FOR AILING AND HEALTHY HEARTS

A Jove Book / published by arrangement with
the author

PRINTING HISTORY
Eleven previous paperback printings

Jove edition / October 1977
Sixth printing / May 1983

All rights reserved.
Copyright © 1969 by Wilfrid E. Shute with Harald J. Taub
This book may not be reproduced in whole or in part,
by mimeograph or any other means, without permission.
For information address: Jove Publications, Inc.,
200 Madison Avenue, New York, N.Y. 10016.

ISBN: 0-515-07512-4

Library of Congress Catalog Card Number: 71-104177

Jove books are published by Jove Publications, Inc.,
200 Madison Avenue, New York, N.Y. 10016.
The words "A JOVE BOOK" and the "J" with sunburst
are trademarks belonging to Jove Publications, Inc.

PRINTED IN THE UNITED STATES OF AMERICA

CONTENTS

INTRODUCTION: *Why Vitamin E?* 7
1. *Alpha Tocopherol* 13
2. *Coronary Occlusion* 25
3. *Angina Pectoris* 43
4. *Ischemic Heart Disease* 51
5. *Rheumatic Fever and Acute Rheumatic Heart Disease* 61
6. *Chronic Rheumatic Heart Disease* 71
7. *The Electrocardiogram* 87
8. *High Blood Pressure* 91
9. *Congenital Heart Disease* 97
10. *Peripheral Vascular Disease* 107
11. *Varicose Veins* 117
12. *Thrombophlebitis* 125
13. *Arterial Thrombi* 133
14. *Indolent Ulcer* 137
15. *Diabetes* 143
16. *Kidney Disease* 151
17. *Burns* 163
18. *Vitamin E Ointment* 171
19. *Tailoring the Dose* 175
20. *Vitamin E on the Moon* 187
21. *Estrogen and Antagonists* 191
22. *Hopeful Horizons* 195
23. *What of the Future?* 201
BIBLIOGRAPHY 203
INDEX 208

INTRODUCTION

WHY VITAMIN E?

WITH WELL OVER A MILLION people a year dying of heart disease in the United States alone, you will not be surprised to read that coronary thrombosis — the major cause of heart attack death — is the greatest single killer in the world today. What you may find very surprising, however, is that coronary thrombosis was unknown as a disease entity in 1900 and apparently hardly existed at that time. Indeed, three cases were reported by Dr. George Dock in 1896, (1) but his reported findings of clots in coronary arteries were not corroborated by other investigators. It was not until 1912 that Herrick (2) in Chicago reported six cases and medical practitioners began to be aware of coronary thrombosis as a possibility.

Dr. Paul Dudley White writes: (3) ". . . when I graduated from medical school in 1911, I had never heard of coronary thrombosis, which is one of the chief threats to life in the United States and Canada today—an astonishing development in one's own lifetime! There can be no doubt but that coronary heart disease has reached epidemic proportions in the United States, where it is now responsible for more than 50 per cent of all deaths. . . .

"The truth is, an ever-increasing number of young men are being struck down before the age of 40 (including a large number of physicians) at the time when they are most needed by their families and when they are prepared to make their greatest contribution to society."

Is there even a remote possibility that the physicians of 50 years ago were both so ignorant and incurious as to be utterly unaware of tens or hundreds of thousands of coronary thromboses occurring before their eyes? Of all possibilities that would seem to be the least likely. In fact some of the most acute and observant pathologists in American medical history were active at this time! It is by far more reasonable to assume that 50 years ago, or any time before then, coronary thrombosis simply was not occurring often enough to constitute any kind of observable disease entity.

We must then ask ourselves, in the light of what we know about this major killer, what changes have occurred in the general conditions of life. What has so recently made people, formerly immune to clots in the coronary arteries, now so very susceptible?

There are many theories, of course. No other disease except cancer has ever provoked so many somewhat plausible, contradictory and unhelpful ideas about causation and prevention. Heart attacks have been blamed on stress and strain, on overexertion, on the fast pace of modern living, on soft drinking water, on hard drinking water, and, of course, on diets rich in animal fats. Among the prominent and more widely held theories, each of these ideas has its own kind of plausibility. Yet with each and every one it can be shown that the same condition was present in the lives of all or many people prior to 1900, but did not cause coronary thrombosis.

Without attempting any complicated statistical proofs, let us simply consider what is obvious about these theories.

While we tend to think of modern living as being conducted at a faster pace, the speed is really more an attribute of our machines than it is of our own lives. We can drive 60 miles an hour, but the stress and strain of traveling 60 miles is infinitely less in driving a car than it was in traveling the same distance in a jolting stage coach threatened by robbers and hostile Indians, or than traveling the same distance on horseback or on foot along bad roads with danger threatening from behind every tree. Before the turn of the century there was more stress involved in caring for larger families on lower earnings; an employee was unprotected before the whims of his boss and knew that if he lost a job it might take months, years, or forever to find another. Even savings were relatively unsafe in banks that failed without warning. Actually, there are very few stresses today that were not present in prethrombotic times.

Dr. Howard B. Sprague of Boston, a former president of the American Heart Association, has stated that "one man's stress is just another man's challenge" and probably has little to do with heart disease.

If our ancestors could live on isolated farms threatened by Indian raids and not get coronaries, stress can hardly be bad for the heart.

Overexertion, like shoveling snow after a blizzard, would be a joke to our forebears, who wrestled horse-drawn plows or worked 12 hard hours a day in factories. True, men do have heart attacks while shoveling snow, but for the causation, except the immediate provocation, we must look elsewhere.

Soft water and hard water, of course, have not changed appreciably. There is no doubt that 50 years ago, 80 or 100 years ago or as far back as you want to go, some people drank hard water and some drank soft, and none of them developed a coronary thrombosis.

Even when it comes to the animal-fat theory, whose adherents are world-wide and whose numbers are legion, there are obvious weaknesses that only need pointing out.

In the American diet it can be shown that the number of foods containing animal or saturated fats has increased greatly, but it can also be shown that in times past people ate all the animal fat available to them. They did not trim their meats. They ate more fried foods than are eaten today. Billions of people subsisted for their entire lives on types of meat with names like "fatback" — and they were not affected with coronary thrombosis. Actually, the intake of animal fat in the American diet has, over the past 15 years, been reduced to approximately one-third of what it was, while, far from decreasing, the coronary rate has gone up every year. During this same period, the intake of animal fats in Canada was relatively unchanged. Yet, although the average Canadian ate three times as much as his American counterpart, the incidence of coronary thrombosis in Canada leveled off, came to a halt, and began to decrease during that same period.

An interesting study of myocardial infarction (heart attack caused by shutting off of the blood supply to the heart by a coronary artery obstruction and consequent death of heart muscle tissue) was reported by Dr. S. L. Malhotra (4) of Bombay, India. He made an illuminating comparison between natives of North India (the Punjab) and those of the South. Natives of the Punjab, he showed, have a fat intake that is largely of animal origin and is eight to 19 times as great as that of the Southerners. But the prevalence of myocardial infarction in Southern India is seven times greater than in the Punjab.

There is much evidence to suggest that there is no relationship between dietary fat and coronary artery disease, although the theory still has its adherents. Similarly, the commonly held relationship between arteriosclerosis and coronary thrombosis may have no validity. Indeed, Morris (5) in England in 1951 demonstrated that in the year 1910 there was more coronary artery atherosclerosis than there is now. Yet, there was little or no coronary thrombosis at that time.

For a very good specific example let us consider the chairman of the Diet-Heart Committee of the American Medical Association, who was scheduled to present to the annual A.M.A. meeting in June, 1967, his recommendation for a very expensive long-term evaluation of the restriction of animal fats in the diet. He, himself, had followed his own recommended low fat regimen for years, had kept slim and exercised frequently, and in all ways followed his own "authoritative" advice on how to prevent heart attacks. He was unable to attend that June, 1967 meeting because he was in hospital recovering from a coronary thrombosis!

Of course, coronary thrombosis as such is not the only form of heart disease. Atherosclerotic changes causing the coronary artery to narrow bring a decrease in blood supply to the heart muscle, which, in turn, leads to gradual changes in the heart. Eventually, there is decreased tolerance to stress or to exertion or excitement, leading to pain in the chest, shortness of breath, or both.

Elevated blood pressure leads to increased strain on the walls of blood vessels, to an accelerated rate of tissue damage, and to an increased possibility of cerebral artery, coronary artery, or peripheral artery insufficiency. The advent of new and effective antihypertensive drugs has brought about a marked improvement in the life expectancy of such patients in the last 15 years. Acute rheumatic fever, which is often preventable by antibiotic treatment of the preceding tonsillitis or pharyngitis, is actually on the decrease.

The fact remains that heart-disease deaths have doubled since 1945, far outstripping the growth in population and amounting today to more than one million deaths a year in the United States alone. By far the major cause of such deaths is coronary thrombosis, which occurs frequently even when there is no atherosclerosis.

Is there, then, a more rational explanation than the animal fat-atherosclerosis theory to explain why a disease entity that did not occur prior to 1910 has become a greater ravager of human life than any plague recorded in history?

There is an explanation so simple that it would automatically be suspect had its truth not already been demonstrated in clinical practice of more than 20 years involving many thousands of patients. I have found in my own practice that alpha tocopherol (vitamin E) is, in addition to its other properties, which will be described herein, a superb antithrombin in the bloodstream. Not only will vitamin E dissolve clots, but circulating in the blood of a healthy individual will prevent thrombi from forming.

Historically, it is irrefutable that when new and more efficient milling methods were introduced into the manufacture of wheat flour, those methods permitting for the first time the complete stripping away of the highly perishable wheat germ, the diet of Western man lost its only significant source of vitamin E. Flour milling underwent this great change around the turn of the century, and it became general around 1910. The amount of vitamin E in the diet was greatly reduced, and with the loss of this natural antithrombin, coronary thrombosis appeared on the scene.

The result of the removal of our major, naturally occurring, circulating antithrombin then explains our present predicament quite fully. The failure of all other methods is apparent from the following statistics of the Metropolitan Life Insurance Company. A "slight increase" was recorded yet again for 1968 in "diseases of the heart, which currently account for nearly two-fifths of all deaths in the United States. The mortality rate for the ischemic type of heart disease, mainly coronary, increased by about three per cent."

Other methods having failed, the time has come when the medical profession must adopt a method of proven success, basically sound, scientifically and abundantly verified by surgeons, physicians, and scientists the world over. As will be apparent in succeeding chapters, this process has already begun in many medical centers.

This book will enable any physician willing to find a better treatment for his cardiac cases to use alpha tocopherol therapy in the ways I have found most successful in my own practice and to learn for himself what vitamin E can or cannot do for the human heart.

WILFRID E. SHUTE
Port Credit, Ontario

CHAPTER 1. *ALPHA TOCOPHEROL*

IT IS SURELY ONE OF THE TRAGedies of modern medicine that the world's first knowledge of vitamin E grew out of the discovery that deficiency in some hitherto unknown food element would reduce the fertility of rats. Even while vitamin E was still being studied and isolated, its initial association with the sexual function made it fascinating to popular medical writers and irresistible to quacks. It was entirely predictable that the vitamin would soon be seized on for useless treatments for impotence and other sexual disorders.

What is tragic is that the medical profession, while feeling a distaste for quack use of the vitamin and properly trying to explode the mythology growing up around it, lost sight of the legitimate need for the vitamin and that, ballyhoo aside, it might be put to valuable therapeutic use. It is probably too much to expect of human beings, but had doctors been able simultaneously to condemn the fakery and accept the growing body of scientific evidence of what vitamin E is good for and how it can be used, literally millions of premature deaths could have been avoided in the period between 1922, when alpha tocopherol was first isolated by Evans and Bishop (6) and also by Sure (7), and the present day.

Clearly and unmistakably alpha tocopherol is a highly effective antithrombin in the bloodstream, yet one which does not induce hemorrhage, suffers from none of the drawbacks of the anticoagulants that are commonly used, and consequently may be used indefinitely without danger. As such, it should be known to every doctor who ever has to treat any type of thrombosis.

Alpha tocopherol has other qualities as well, but it is its antithrombin activity that distinguishes it from six other associated tocopherols in the foods containing the vitamin. Since 1945 when it was established that in the vitamin E complex only the alpha tocopherol is biologically active as an antithrombin, the strength of vitamin E preparations has been rated pharmacologically in terms of their alpha tocopherol content. One milligram of alpha tocopherol is equal to one international unit of vitamin E activity. To most scientists today, vitamin E and alpha tocopherol are the same substance, even though the other tocopherols of the vitamin E complex are not entirely inactive, but do possess antioxidant properties. Pure alpha tocopherol was synthesized 1938 by Karrer (8) and has been widely available for use since 1941.

Our interest in vitamin E really began in 1933 with the evaluation and extension of an empirical treatment for the menstrual difficulties dysmenorrhea and menorrhagia devised by our father, Dr. R. James Shute, of Windsor, Ontario, Canada. Our father's use of thyroid extract, a treatment he originated that is now widely used, showed a certain similarity in its clinical effect to the then known properties of vitamin E with which Dr. Evan Shute had recently been working. This led to a research project, under a grant from the Banting Institute, which in turn led to a chemical method for qualitative and rough quantitative determination of the estrogen level in the circulating blood. This in turn led to evidence that both thyroid extract and vitamin E were antagonists to estrogen, though the mode of action of the antagonism was different in the two substances.

Further investigation led to successes in the treatment of threatened abortion, the prevention of *abruptio placenta*, a cause of miscarriage in pregnancy, and prevention of the toxemias of late pregnancy, as well as other difficult conditions found in a specialist's practice in obstetrics and gynecology. In much of this work, Dr. Evan Shute was joined by his father, Dr. James Shute, and later by the author.

During the early days of our experience with vitamin E, we were able to obtain a potent wheat-germ-oil product and to maintain its potency for some weeks by refrigeration. Using this product, Dr. Evan Shute obtained complete relief of severe angina pectoris in one patient. We now know that this one patient was unique in that he responded to an unusually low concentration of the alpha tocopherol. Fortunately, also, he was one of the few people who could tolerate, without nausea, the taste of this product in large quantity. An attempt on the part of the author to duplicate this accomplishment on similar patients failed, and we discontinued all efforts in this direction for some time.

Meanwhile, research on the use of vitamin E was continued in other fields with considerable success until some nine years later when, as a result of the research grant to a university student for summer work, our interest in the use of the vitamin for cardiovascular treatment was reawakened. This student, now Dr. Floyd Skelton, was casting about for a suitable research project and approached Dr. Evan Shute for suggestions. As a result, a project was initiated using estrogen to induce thrombocytopenic purpura in dogs and, thereafter, curing and preventing the same hemorrhagic disease with vitamin E. The design of the study was a logical extension of my brother's original findings that the two substances, estrogen and vitamin E, are antagonists.

The experiments demonstrated conclusively that easy bruising and prolonged bleeding, with low platelet count, in the dog could be induced by estrogen and cured by vitamin E. Similarly, dogs protected by vitamin E could not be made purpuric by estrogen.

The real turning point in the discovery of the value of vitamin E in heart disease was the direct result of the application of the knowledge gained by Skelton with these dogs. The first human case of severe thrombocytopenic purpura on which it was tried was that of a man in deep congestive heart failure. His condition was the only reason he was considered a fit subject for the trial. Again, unusual luck accompanied the venture, since he also responded rapidly and completely to what we now consider a threshold, or often inadequate, level of the drug, namely 200 units. His congestive failure cleared up before the purpura disappeared. This established two characteristics of vitamin E treatment: one, that the dosage level, as calculated from Skelton's experience with dogs, was 20 to 50 times that suggested for the substance up to that time, and two, that it was the alpha fraction of vitamin E which was the active portion.

Many months later, when because of the excessive cost of this synthetic alpha tocopherol, we switched to the natural form as manufactured by Distillation Products Industries in Rochester, New York, the clinical results were exactly comparable when only the alpha fraction of the oil was equated to that of the synthetic alpha tocopherol product.

The fact that this first patient was a cardiac cripple being treated by Dr. Arthur Vogelsang and that Dr. Evan Shute, being an obstetrician and gynecologist, had few, if any, cardiac patients, brought the author into the project of further investigation of the effect of vitamin E in cardiac disease.

The first patients were maintained on their previous regimens with the one exception that now 300 units of alpha tocopherol daily were added. Improvement, when obtained, could then be attributed only to the one substance.

In all this investigative work, with the exception of the one patient successfully treated in 1936, Dr. Evan Shute served as guide and co-ordinator. He has continued his very successful obstetrical and gynecological work, while taking time to assist with its extension to such peripheral blood-vessel problems as arteriosclerotic changes in the extremities, failing circulation and gangrene of Buerger's Disease, diabetic gangrene, etc. Cardiac treatment became the province of Drs. Vogelsang and the author. Separately and together the cardiovascular aspect, in all its variations and ramifications, was investigated and for nearly 25 years has been the exclusive interest and occupation of the author.

The number of patients whose treatment I have supervised personally or through other doctors working at The Shute

Institute now exceeds 30,000. This is somewhere in the realm of five times as many cardiovascular patients as seen by any other living doctor.

This work, widely published in medical journals since 1945, has stimulated investigators in our own and other countries, and there is now, as will be shown later, a very large bibliography available for those interested in its clinical application — the purpose of this book.

By now it is possible to say with complete assurance that alpha tocopherol is a thoroughly tried and tested therapeutic agent, unusually successful in its results and with its effects so well defined that it can be used with precision by any competent physician.

Given carefully produced alpha tocopherol of known potency in terms of international units, it is a simple matter to prove its effectiveness in combatting cardiovascular disease. This can be demonstrated in 48 to 96 hours in a case of acute inflammation of the kidney (nephritis), acute rheumatic fever, or acute thrombophlebitis. Such cases, treated as soon as the diagnosis can be established, will be, by all criteria, laboratory and clinical, completely cured in two to four days! Such a potent drug, if it had no other value than in the treatment of such cases, is an absolute necessity in the armamentarium of every doctor whatever his specialty or type of practice.

The action of alpha tocopherol has been extensively investigated and its chemical use extensively confirmed. Up to 1961 there were 391 articles supporting the use of alpha tocopherol in cardiovascular-renal diseases in the medical literature written by 668 clinicians and investigators from 35 countries. The volume of papers published since has more than doubled, and this substantiates the statement made above that the effectiveness of alpha tocopherol in this field of medicine has now been thoroughly established. All that remains is to have every doctor use it whenever indicated.

Like all useful therapy, it requires a thorough knowledge of its modes of application. Given a good product, the dosage must be adequate to control the specific condition. For example, in treating coronary disease, the dosage range is around 600 to 800 units daily or more. If patients with chronic rheumatic heart disease are given this same dosage, the majority will become dramatically and rapidly much improved, but will then worsen; if this dosage level is continued the majority will develop rapid cardiac decompensation with failure and death. On the other hand, a relatively low initial dose gradually increased will usually lead to very worthwhile improvement not obtainable in any other way.

Just as the physician can adequately control the sugar in the diabetic only when he matches the dosage of insulin to the individual patient's needs, so the doctor using alpha tocopherol must know the dosage range and then tailor it to his patient's requirement.

Fortunately, in practice alpha tocopherol can be effectively combined with any other known treatment. There are virtually only three known, commonly used drugs with which alpha tocopherol is incompatible — inorganic iron, mineral oil, and female sex hormone. Iron leaches it out, and if iron must be given for anemia, for example, it must be kept from coming in direct contact with it. This can be done therapeutically by having the patient take all his alpha tocopherol in one dose and all his iron eight to 12 hours later.

Vegetable oils dissolve alpha tocopherol but readily release it in the body, while mineral oil dissolves it but does not readily release it.

Estrogen is an antagonist to alpha tocopherol, is very rarely necessary in cardiovascular cases, and should be avoided whenever possible. Its use makes it very difficult to estimate the amount of alpha tocopherol the patient is using. Alpha tocopherol has an action similar to that of digitalis on the hypoxic (oxygen deficient) heart. For this reason any digitalis given is more effective in the patient on alpha tocopherol than in one without alpha tocopherol. In most cases, the dosage of digitalis used should be no more than a half of the usual therapeutic dose and may be much less.

With these exceptions any other indicated drug may be

used along with alpha tocopherol. Nitroglycerine, the antihypertensive drugs, and the diuretics can safely be used as adjunct therapy, for example, and indeed seem to be more effective because of the simultaneous use of alpha tocopherol.

The original work on the use of alpha tocopherol in cardiovascular disease was carried out by Dr. Floyd Skelton, then a medical student, and three doctors, Evan Shute, Arthur Vogelsang, and the author. The work of Ochsner and the definitive work of Zierler, *et al* (9) was done later. The product originally used was synthetic, and the results were excellent. Later, when the natural product became available, we were again fortunate that the product selected was properly assayed and labeled. The results were completely comparable, one international unit of the synthetic equal to one international unit of the natural product, irrespective of how much or how little of the other tocopherols were present in the capsule. However, studies made by biochemists at Distillation Products Industries have found about 30 per cent greater biological activity in natural alpha tocopherol.

There is now such a very large number of scientific reports on the efficacy of alpha tocopherol in the treatment of cardiovascular and renal diseases that there should be no longer any hesitancy about its use. The only ones qualified to discuss its properties are those who have used it. There are, of course, no other such safe and potent forms of treatment available.

Unfortunately, the original papers dealing with the use of anticoagulants were widely circulated, and that treatment was rapidly and universally adopted. It is remarkable that it took nearly 12 years and many thousands of cases before it was discovered that the drug was probably useless and, of course, highly dangerous. By this time hospital labs had trained technicians to do the necessary blood analyses, and it is hard now to abandon the treatment. The same applies to the cholesterol theory and, of course, to "bed rest." As early as 1952 Dr. Samuel Levine was able to lower the death rate of acute coronary thrombosis cases from approximately 40 to 60 to 9.9 per cent, merely by taking the patient out of bed as soon as his pain had subsided and putting him in a comfortable chair with arms and a seat which supported the buttocks and thighs evenly. Yet for years after the inefficacy of the regimen had been irrefutably demonstrated, bed rest, abstention from exertion and excitement, retirement, and an afternoon nap were advocated for patients who had survived their initial attack.

There has been a similar lag between knowledge of the effectiveness of alpha tocopherol and its use.

Mode of Action of Alpha Tocopherol

Following recovery from a coronary occlusion, the patient usually, but by no means always, develops the intense chest pain known as angina pectoris. In many cases, angina pectoris has preceded the onset of the so-called attack.

Similarly, in patients in whom there has been no history of occlusion and no clinical or electrocardiographic evidence of such an episode, angina pectoris develops gradually due to narrowing of the coronary arteries and the consequent diminution of blood supply to the heart muscle — the myocardium.

Commonly in diabetes mellitus of some years' duration, narrowing of the interior channel — the lumen of arteries in brain, eye, heart, kidney, or the extremities, occurs. There is always in the diabetic female, and nearly always in the male, such narrowing to a degree greater than that expected for that age group.

Narrowing of the arteries in the legs occurs in many older people and also occurs along with episodes of spasm and thrombosis in those with Buerger's Disease.

In all such cases the action of alpha tocopherol, which diminishes or relieves these symptoms, depends upon its power to decrease the oxygen need of the involved tissues. In most cases, this decrease will be marked; in many, very much worthwhile; in a few, not sufficient to warrant its further use for this purpose — the relief of pain. Of course, many factors are involved. A few are:

1. The blood vessels, while following a generally typical basic pattern, show many variations in all people. (Thomas N. James in his book "Anatomy of the Coronary Arteries" has demonstrated these variations beautifully. The coronary circulation, arterial and venous, was injected with colored solutions of vinylite dissolved in acetone with kaolin and the heart muscle eroded away in concentrated hydrochloric acid.) Since these vessels must carry the alpha tocopherol to the affected myocardium, the size, number, and degree of proliferation of small arteries must affect the quantity of the active medication that can reach the area supplied by these vessels.

2. The degree of utilization and the speed and degree of excretion of alpha tocopherol, as well as the amount ingested, also affect the amount of active medication reaching the deprived area.

3. Of great importance is the individual response to alpha tocopherol. Houchin and Mattill (10) showed that in anoxic (oxygen deficient) isolated heart muscle the addition of alpha tocopherol decreased the oxygen need by some 50 to 250 per cent. This explains the wide variations in response in individual patients. Obviously, the man who obtains a 250 per cent decrease in oxygen need will never thereafter run out of oxygen whatever his initial condition, while the man who obtains only 50 per cent reduction will be only partially helped.

This ability of alpha tocopherol to reduce oxygen need, and thereby increase exercise tolerance has been demonstrated in normal animals, racing greyhounds, race horses, and in humans in baseball, hockey, figure skating, and swimming.

At least part of this demonstrable effect derives from the well-established fact that vitamin E is a biological antioxidant. By preventing premature and undesirable oxidation of lipids in the bloodstream, it keeps available to the tissues a higher proportion of the oxygen taken into the blood.

The second action of alpha tocopherol of major importance

in cardiovascular disease has been mentioned previously — its ability to dissolve fresh thrombi and to prevent the occurrence of thrombosis. The patient suffering from the results of a previous thrombosis in coronary artery, vein, or peripheral vessel will thus be almost, though not quite completely, protected from a recurrence.

The results of these two major actions of alpha tocopherol, therefore, lead to marked clinical improvement in:

- Fresh coronary thrombosis.
- Cases which have survived coronary thrombosis without alpha tocopherol treatment.
- Angina pectoris due to coronary artery narrowing.
- Fresh thrombophlebitis.
- Recurring acute and subacute thrombophlebitis.
- Buerger's Disease.
- Peripheral vascular arteriosclerosis and insufficiency, including intermittent claudication.
- Diabetic and arteriosclerotic early gangrene.
- Diabetic and arteriosclerotic retinitis.
- To a much lesser degree, results of cerebral artery thrombosis or embolus.

There are other specific actions of alpha tocopherol which are of importance, but which may either apply more particularly to a specific situation or else occur gradually and whose results are less obvious or dramatic.

In acute, early stages of rheumatic fever the ability of alpha tocopherol to return abnormal capillary permeability to normal, as well as its oxygen-sparing characteristic, seems to prevent specific damage to the tissues concerned. An acutely ill patient may be in every detectable sense normal in 48 to 96 hours and will not develop sequelae.

It is this same action of the restoration of normal capillary permeability that saves the kidney from irreparable damage in fresh acute nephritis. The edema of the kidney, with the resulting swelling inside the inelastic capsule and the pressure on the glomeruli characteristic of the disease, is prevented or decreased, thus preserving the glomeruli until the other actions of alpha tocopherol overcome the disease. An acute nephritis will characteristically be cured by all available tests in 48 to 96 hours. This is why immediate treatment with alpha tocopherol of rheumatic fever and nephritis must be initiated at the first definite signs of the disease.

Alpha tocopherol increases the extent and the speed of the opening up of collateral circulation, and this is of great importance in the treatment of intermittent claudication and of chronic thrombophlebitis, indeed of any condition involving the peripheral circulation, venous or arterial. Since the collateral circulation in the brain and heart is poorly developed by contrast to the peripheral circulation, its action in this respect is much less obvious and is slow to appear, as well as hard to evaluate.

Finally, the effect of alpha tocopherol on scar tissue is of utmost importance in wounds and burns. Wide areas of burned tissue will heal and become epithelialized without the inevitable contraction. The scars following alpha tocopherol topically and orally administered are like no other scars ever seen. In many cases skin grafting need no longer be indicated, and in other cases the amount of skin grafting can be greatly reduced.

CHAPTER 2. *CORONARY OCCLUSION*

DURING THE CHRISTMAS HOLIDAYS in 1967, I was called to attend a neighbor who had suffered a severe heart attack.

On a clear, cold day he had been out with his son playing ice hockey, a popular sport in Canada. While playing he suddenly experienced severe pain in the mid-sternal region of the chest. He knew something serious was happening, called his son away from the game, removed his skates, and assisted by the boy made his way to their car to drive home.

They lived only a few blocks away, but before they reached home he had to stop the car to vomit and was barely able to drive the last block to his house.

He was able to make his way into the split-level house and up a small flight of stairs, but the attack became so severe he collapsed before he could negotiate the final 15 feet to his bed.

I tried to relieve his pain as he lay there and moved him to the hospital by ambulance as soon as possible. In spite of several doses of morphine administered subcutaneously and intravenous dilators, he remained in pain for nearly 24 hours. Vitamin E (alpha tocopherol), 1,600 units daily, was started immediately with the full dosage given the evening of admission. Experience has shown that when treatment is started immediately after the attack, the recovery is more rapid and more complete and the electrocardiogram returns to or toward normal more rapidly than when it is begun later. There is, therefore, no time to waste.

This man's electrocardiogram showed the usual changes of an anterior myocardial infarction involving all precordial leads and, therefore, presumably due to a thrombus in a major branch of the left anterior descending coronary or the artery itself.

I am reporting this case in some detail for two reasons. The first is to point out the incompleteness and the consequent inadequacy of any advice on how to prevent heart attacks, no matter how well-intentioned or how professional, that does not include vitamin E. When he was well on the road to recovery, this patient and neighbor, while recuperating in the hospital, watching television, reading newspapers and paperback novels, one day expressed himself vehemently to me on the subject of the "clean life." This was one patient who had not neglected himself, at least not deliberately. He had for years carefully watched his weight and diet, retaining a trim figure free of any hint of obesity. He had made it a point to exercise daily. Regardless of the weather, which can get prohibitively severe in Ontario, he had taken a two- to three-mile walk every night. Even more remarkable, this man had never smoked, did not drink alcohol, and made it a point to go to bed early and sleep eight hours every night. Even when he went to business conventions, he never stayed at the convention hotel but always got separate accommodations so that he could avoid involvement in the late hours and carousing typical of such meetings. And the net result, he told me bitterly, was that he had a heart attack anyway. I explained to my patient that while I cannot dispute the strong opinions of many important cardiologists that such a regimen has good preventive value, none of these measures can prevent thrombosis if the bloodstream is deficient in the antithrombin content that should naturally be there. As soon as his antithrombin level dropped below the critical level, I told him, a coronary thrombosis was imminent no matter how sensibly he lived. And that, I explained, was why I was treating him with alpha tocopherol, which is the chief and, perhaps, the only natural antithrombin in the human body as Zierler *et al* (10) have pointed out.

My second reason for describing this particular case history is another conversation I had with this patient during the three weeks he was in hospital. He asked me how often I heard good things about myself in the hospital and told me that, during his time there, three nurses on his floor, none of them on his case, had come to tell him that he was lucky to have me for his doctor. Each of them said to him that my treatment was totally different from what any other doctors in the hospital used — but that my patients live!

There can be no question about the superb antithrombin activity of alpha tocopherol or that an antithrombin, without side effects and particularly that will *not* induce hemorrhaging, is of importance beyond measure in the treatment of coronary occlusion. As accepted an authority and as respected a surgeon as Alton Ochsner, M.D., has demonstrated that neither roughening nor damage of the lining of a blood vessel is necessary for the formation of a thrombus, as occurs in the veins of the leg after surgery or childbirth. Ochsner also has found through a long career as a surgeon that alpha tocopherol is the best prophylaxis, as well as treatment, for this condition. Twenty full years ago, in 1949, Ochsner reported the ability of alpha tocopherol to dissolve and harmlessly remove freshly formed thrombi in the large veins of the legs. In 1964 (July 23) he reported in the *New England Journal of Medicine* that he had been using alpha tocopherol routinely to prevent venous thrombosis; and four years later in 1968 he reported again that, because of this routine prophylaxis, he had no trouble with pulmonary emboli, the breaking loose in the veins of clots which are then carried through the heart and into the vessels of the lungs.

It may well be asked, if both the antithrombin properties and lack of danger of alpha tocopherol are well known and established, why is it not more widely used?

One answer to that question is an unreasonably prolonged natural lag which seems to occur in medical practice between the announcement of important discoveries and their general adoption. A typical example is the enormously important discovery by Dr. Samuel Levine (12), of Boston, that he could greatly increase the recovery rate among his heart attack patients by abandoning the concept of bed rest and preferentially, as soon as possible, getting his patients out of bed and seating them upright in a chair. It is a simple enough change in treatment. Dr. Levine is recognized as a leader among cardiologists. Yet 16 years after he had reported his improved technique, I was still the only doctor in Toronto to employ it. Small wonder that the nurses, at least, have noticed that my methods are different from those of my immediate colleagues.

In the case of the particular patient I have described, as soon as he was out of pain, 24 hours after his admission to the hospital, he was placed in a comfortable armchair with a comfortable seat which did not put undue pressure across the backs of his legs at the front of the seat, a precaution that should be carefully observed. Like all other patients so treated, he was left there until he complained of fatigue, all day if possible. He was allowed to go to the bathroom from the second day of hospitalization.

With this treatment, patients do not feel ill, do not lose strength, and are saved a great deal of mental anguish and depression. They are not aware that you may still be fighting for their lives, and even this psychic advantage can be a great one. This particular patient was discharged from hospital in three weeks. During the next three weeks at home he gradually resumed normal activities, worked at some paper work from his office, and eight weeks after his occlusion was able to return to work.

There is an interesting postscript to this case. This man is a highly placed executive in one of the largest tire manufacturing companies. The company has just been sold a package deal by an enterprising medical group and has arranged for a complete check-up of all its senior executives. This patient, 16 months after his acute coronary occlusion, has just had exhaustive tests of every kind, a multitude of X-rays, intravenous dyes and, finally, a most thorough heart check-up. His resting electrocardiogram and his several electrocardiograms taken after the Master Step Test are all completely normal. He was the only one of that company's executives able to do the complete test!

I have now initiated this treatment in three hospitals. In each of them, at first, there was extreme apprehension and alarm among the nursing staff and a great reluctance to carry out my instructions. It was only by invoking the great name and reputation of Dr. Samuel Levine that I was able to get the nurses to cooperate. Yet the improvement is so much faster and so marked that each time, on about the fifth to tenth day of treatment, one or more graduate nurses has suggested that the patient couldn't possibly have had a heart attack or he would not be so well so fast. Since so treating the first two or three patients in each hospital, I have had the most complete cooperation from the nurses.

In a practice of cardiology that has probably been the most extensive in the Western Hemisphere, I have become completely convinced that the combination of Levine's armchair treatment and the earliest possible initiation of alpha tocopherol therapy make up a regimen that salvages more patients than any other currently available treatment by far while greatly reducing the extent of damage to the heart.

It is probably well to make it clear at this point that during the past 22 years the author has been called on to treat or supervise the treatment of more than 30,000 cardiovascular patients and may be presumed at this point, to have acquired some knowledge that is more than theoretical. These patients have come from every state in the U.S., every province of Canada, England, Ireland, Australia, New Zealand, Switzerland, India, and the Isle of Capri. They have all received conventional treatment for their cardiac conditions and obviously have all had residual symptoms and reason to fear another attack, or they would not have made their long journeys to Ontario to seek a better treatment. Many of these patients have themselves been physicians. In most cases they have been physicians who have recognized the logic of alpha tocopherol treatment yet have lacked the courage to administer this reasonable therapy to their own patients because of what they consider rightly or wrongly an oppressive and censorial professional climate in which they practice.

Such doctors have been pleased and, in some cases,

amazed at the effectiveness of the basically simple treatment they have received. Thus the reader should be aware that, whether it is generally admitted or not, alpha tocopherol therapy is not merely the province of a small group of physicians working in isolation in a Canadian province, but has been put to the test under the most severe and practical conditions by thousands of physicians and has been found highly effective.

Since so many of my patients come from distant places and must clearly be able to travel before coming to me, it is apparent that most of them who have had coronary occlusions are seen weeks or months after treatment elsewhere. Not having been seen in the acute stage, they cannot be said to represent a cross-section of coronary cases. They are nevertheless a better than usual sampling in that they have all been first diagnosed and treated as coronaries by other perfectly competent doctors, usually unknown to me, and then have been diagnostically confirmed by me. The possibility of diagnostic error is thus reduced virtually to zero.

In some of the patients there is evidence of congestive failure or peripheral edema. Some are frankly in the last stages of circulatory failure. Most of them present simply the usual symptoms of angina pectoris (severe chest pain occurring in sudden, acute attacks because of insufficient blood supply to the heart) or dsypnea (difficulty in breathing) or both, brought on episodically by exertion or excitement. No patient, no matter how difficult or hopeless the case may seem, is ever refused treatment. Substantial and worthwhile relief is obtained by 80 to 85 percent of them.

Coronary occlusion is a general term describing various forms of disease involving the coronary artery which lead to complete blockage of the arterial passage — in effect, obliteration of the lumen. The commonest form of occlusion by far is the formation of a thrombus — a clot — in the artery itself. On occasion, a calcified plaque that has formed in the arterial wall will tear loose at its upper edge and block off the passage of blood, completely obliterating the lumen. It is also presumably possible for a small clot, or a portion broken off from the larger thrombus in the left ventricle of the heart, to find its way into the coronary artery at its point of origin just behind the cusps of the aortic valve and, upon being carried into a small branch of the artery, close it off. Finally atheromatous plaques — the formations on arterial walls that constitute the disease entity known as atherosclerosis — may be so large and situated in such a way that, by their developing growth, they reach a point in which the lumen is completely closed off.

Whichever the cause, the sudden occlusion is usually — though not always — a catastrophe. By the total closing off of a coronary artery or even a branch of a coronary artery, an area of heart muscle is completely deprived of blood and thus receives no oxygen. The tissue that is so affected dies. The area of myocardium that dies in this way for lack of oxygen is called a myocardial infarct, just as the condition is known as a myocardial infarction.

The heart and brain are the two organs susceptible to this type of sudden disaster. Except in the heart and brain, there are extensive networks of communicating vessels joining larger vessels to still larger vessels, very much the way a tree branches with each branch putting out its own network of still smaller branches. Thus in the area of most organs, even large blood vessels can be completely tied off, without serious jeopardy to the life of the tissues that are mainly supplied by the large vessels, if the other smaller vessels in the area are relatively normal.

In the heart and brain, however, the collateral circulation is relatively poor. As a result, the blocking off of a large coronary artery or large branch will always lead to complete deprivation of blood supply to some area of heart muscle. Whether the result is complete or only partial disaster depends very much on the location of the thrombus and how large an area of the myocardium is affected by it. Of great importance also is the integrity of the heart muscle elsewhere in the heart, and this depends on how adequate the coronary blood flow to the balance of the heart is at the moment of occlusion. Obviously, there are many factors involved.

If the insult to the heart is severe, the patient will die instantly as he walks or sits or sleeps. If it is less severe, he may survive to leave the hospital with a degree of damage varying widely in different cases.

The chief symptom of a sudden coronary occlusion, of course, is severe chest pain — usually in the center of the chest anteriorly — and this may be very severe indeed, feeling like a ton weight or often described as if a tight band encircled the chest. However, frank myocardial infarction can occur without involving the chest pain.

"Estimates of the incidence of painless myocardial infarction have varied from 0 to 61 per cent depending upon the author," the Framingham group reported. Twenty-one per cent were considered to be completely free from pain. A man may well die of an acute coronary occlusion without any chest pain.

Often the difference between life and death lies in the amount of collateral circulation to the heart that has been developed. It is only through exercise that the heart gains such an auxiliary blood and oxygen supply.

In the 1930's, stress and strain or physical exertion were thought to be causal in the occurrence of this relatively rare disease of old men, and treatment consisted solely of morphine to allay apprehension and as nearly absolute as possible rest in bed for six weeks or longer. All this has been changed recently, since exertion and excitement have been shown to be unrelated except in a casual way to the onset of this condition. It has been shown that the man who remains physically active has a diminished chance of developing a coronary occlusion, that when he does it is likely to be less severe, and that resumption of physical activity following recovery from the acute phase is probably desirable.

However, it remained for Samuel Levine, who along with Paul Dudley White was one of the first two physicians in the U.S. to specialize in cardiology, to demonstrate conclusively that bed rest was undesirable. In 1952 he published a paper (**12**) in the *Journal of the American Medical Association* with the unscientific title "The Myth of Bed Rest in the Treatment of Coronary Thrombosis." He described the treatment of acute cases by hospitalization in an arm chair for three weeks – the treatment to begin as soon as the initial chest pain was relieved. By this simple method, he was able to demonstrate the reduction of the initial death rate to 9.9 per cent instead of the expected 40 to 60 per cent. In other words, four out of five who would have died with intensive care and absolute bed rest lived in the arm-chair treatment.

It has been made apparent in the previous chapter that there is also some chance of reducing the amount of damage to the heart muscle by dissolution of the clot itself, restoring circulation to the necrotic area, and by preventing any extension or recurrence. Obviously, the sooner this patient starts to take and absorb alpha tocopherol, the better. In the original paper by Dr. Alton Ochsner, on alpha tocopherol as an antithrombin, he stated that in the prevention of clots in the veins of the legs, a dosage of 600 units of alpha tocopherol was effective. This is probably an adequate dosage for most patients. However, some need more, and since there is no laboratory test as yet to determine each patient's exact requirements, we take no chances but start the patient immediately on 1,600 international units a day. Except in special circumstances to be described later, there is no danger—not even any discomfort—in surplus dosage. The only danger lies in using too little.

We treat the initial shock and pain by sufficient morphine and by intravenous, inhalation and oral vasodilators for the quickest possible restoration of circulation. The patient sits up as soon as possible, that point being marked by the cessation of severe pain.

Treatment of the Patient Who Has Survived to Leave the Hospital

Alpha tocopherol is the keystone of the treatment. During the early explorations of its unique value, the first three cardiac patients we treated were in frank failure, all three seriously ill. When alpha tocopherol and alpha tocopherol alone was added to their treatment, all three experienced a marked diuresis, all three lost all or nearly all of their failure, and all three returned to normal activity.

Many thousands of patients later, nearly all my cardiac patients are routinely started on 800 I.U. of alpha tocopherol a day and raised by 200 to 400 I.U. a day at six-week intervals if necessary.

Patients will usually show no effects of treatment for the first five to ten days. Most of them, however, will be free of symptoms of angina pectoris or dyspnea in four to six weeks of treatment. Since alpha tocopherol is apparently an "all or none" substance, the patient either responds in four to six weeks, or he doesn't. If he doesn't the dosage level is raised for the next six weeks, or at six-week intervals until he either responds or is obviously not going to respond. There will be no doubt in the mind of patient or physician in either case, since the effect of the drug is so obvious.

Since there is no toxicity with alpha tocopherol treatment, in the typical cardiac case the only problem is to use enough. It is a peculiarity of this and many drugs that half a dose does not accomplish half a result.

However, although alpha tocopherol is the basic treatment, we now make use of all other available useful drugs to hasten in all possible ways the recovery of patients and to obtain as complete a result as possible. We use diuretics freely as needed, as long as they are needed, hoping that after six to eight weeks they will no longer be necessary. We control the apical rate in auricular fibrillation with digitalis, remembering that diuretics on the one hand and alpha tocopherol on the other potentiate the action of digitalis preparations. We use very little digitalis in the absence of auricular fibrillation—usually none.

A word is needed about hypertension in its relation to coronary occlusion. There are five factors, chiefly, maintaining blood pressure: the volume of the blood, its viscosity, the beating action of the heart, the elasticity of the vessel wall, and the peripheral resistance. Many of the cardiac patients seen have or have had an elevation of blood pressure. Alpha tocopherol in a large dose increases the tone of heart muscle and so tends to increase the blood pressure in those who have had or still do have hypertension. On the other hand, small doses of alpha tocopherol have been shown to decrease the peripheral resistance and so to lower blood pressure. Therefore, in such cases we are careful to control the blood pressure with the modern antihypertensive drugs and usually begin treatment of such patients with a lower dosage level of tocopherol.

This precaution is not necessary in the acute case, since blood pressure falls with the occlusion and the tendency of alpha tocopherol to raise it is a beneficial effect.

In treating the hypertensive patient, if the pressure begins to rise, the drug should be stopped for a day or a day and a half and resumed at a lower level. All the effect of alpha tocopherol is lost in as little as three days, so one must never withdraw it for longer than one or two days once it has achieved the desired result.

Fortunately if the patient does respond, his improvement will continue for months and even years, and his electrocardiogram will often show progressive slow improvement, probably due to the development of increased collateral circulation, for months or years.

There have been so many of these patients treated in the last 22 years. Results, of course, have been quite varied in individual cases. Many patients have survived many years after one or even more occlusions, and there are hundreds who have survived ten to 20 years, some even longer. This, of course, is one of the most gratifying experiences a doctor can have.

Several cases will illustrate the extent of improvement that can be obtained. These are among those who have secured the maximum oxygen-sparing faculty of the drug.

One man, aged 47, following his occlusion was unable to walk a block in the city without severe angina pectoris. After five weeks treatment he rejoined the 48 Highlanders and went on a route march. He was able to walk at a military pace up and down hills without pain.

Another, aged 56, was a farmer. He was completely incapacitated following a coronary occlusion, and a nephew was looking after the farm. About five weeks after beginning treatment, he thought he could help the nephew a little around the barn so one morning harnessed up the team of horses and began to hitch them to a wagon. One of the team, a young horse, became frightened and, with the other one, bolted and began to run away. The patient dug his heels into the ground, see-sawed the reins, and pulled the team to a halt just as they reached the gate. Then he realized what he had done!

At this writing a 61-year-old man and his wife are on a trip around the world.

Twenty years ago this man had a coronary occlusion and apparently was dead on arrival at the hospital. He was brought there by ambulance, given oxygen from the moment the ambulance reached the home. One of the ambulance attendants wanted to practice the use of the oxygen equipment and, since the tank was nearly empty anyway, continued to administer oxygen. The patient began to breathe and survived the attack. A year later he had a second occlusion, was very seriously ill, but refused to go to a hospital. He survived this attack also, but was left a cardiac cripple. A very restless, always active man, he chafed under enforced idleness and came to The Shute Institute for help. This man's recovery is unbelievable in that he not only lives a normal life but delights in building complicated summer cottage structures, stairways over huge rocks, sea-walls of stone and cement, fountains, etc. He has been carrying two pails of cement at a time, all day long, all this past summer, up slopes and stairs to reach places inaccessible by wheelbarrow. He runs a machine shop, operates a small bulldozer, and has no angina pectoris or dyspnea at all.

Of course, these are exceptional cases, though there are many like them. Some patients do not seem to obtain any worthwhile benefits, although in such cases we still recommend continuation of treatment for protection against the recurrence of attack—something of real importance to all such patients.

Here are more case histories: One 65-year-old man was first seen at his cabin overlooking Rabbit Bay in one of the most beautiful lakes of the Canadian North. He had been brought there so he might look out over his favorite section of the North woods as he died. He was sitting up in bed gasping for breath in the last stages of congestive failure, with an abdomen enormously distended with huge liver and what must have been nearly maximum ascites (effusion of serous fluid). His legs were as big as tree trunks.

This man was one of the original settlers in the area, had trapped and sold furs, had lumbered his land, and had been a good neighbor. He was a gregarious and generous Irishman, much beloved by many friends. One of these, a lumber baron and patient of mine, had sought me out at a holiday camp and insisted I see the patient.

He had had two coronary occlusions and after the second one gradually developed congestive failure and was hospitalized in the nearest Northern hospital. Because his condition worsened, he was sent to a large university hospital in Toronto where he spent several weeks. He was returned to the Northern hospital still in congestive failure, and finally his doctor, who knew him well and had cared for his large family for years, suggested that he be taken carefully to his cottage on this beautiful lake with the large picture window overlooking the bay — where I, at the end of a holiday, was brought to him.

Obviously, he was much too ill to move, and I had only three more days left before having to return to my office. Also, I had purposely not brought the tools of my trade with me and had no blood pressure cuff or stethoscope with me. So I explained that the situation was hopeless, that he would need a lot of emergency care, with diuretics, punctures to drain off serum, etc., and that I could not remain to give care to him. His daughter told me she was the office nurse of the family doctor and that she and the rest of the family would do anything for their father. So against my better judgment, we drove 25 miles into town and obtained a blood pressure cuff and stethoscope from the doctor's office, went to the hospital for mercurial diuretics, only to find they had none, then to the various drug stores, all of which but one were closed for the Thursday half-holiday.

My indefatigable lumber baron started to throw his weight around and bullied half the druggists to open up and search for the needed drugs. One had some vitamin E, but no diuretics. Finally, we located a doctor who had three vials — samples — of a pre-World War I mercurial diuretic, and we returned to the cottage to begin treatment.

By shipping up supplies after I returned to practice and by almost daily telephone consultations with the daughter, this patient was successfully treated. Within two weeks, he was out of bed. That fall he cut a road into the bush and supervised cutting and logging operations. The following summer I visited him, and they had to call him in from the lake where he was canoeing. He insisted on paddling us around the bay and insisted on presenting us with our choice of lots from among his 2,000 feet of shoreline. Three years later he built us a cottage on that lot.

I hesitate to add this footnote, but it may interest my profession and highlight our interesting experiences of the early days of vitamin E. Although they attended the same church and frequently met on the steps, his own doctor refused to acknowledge his existence or to speak to him. He had dared to get better!

Female — aged 50 when first seen.

This highly educated, short, obese colored woman was first seen April 13, 1949.

She had suffered an acute coronary occlusion with an anterior myocardial infarct in February of 1948. For the six months before the actual attack she had had considerable angina. She was kept in bed until June of 1948 — a period of four months — so severe was the attack.

When first seen she had angina and dyspnea on exertion, such as climbing stairs, but could slowly walk about six blocks in the city.

On 600 units of alpha tocopherol she lost all angina and dyspnea and returned to her work as a teacher of languages in high school. She retired from teaching in June of 1958 when 68 years old.

Now aged 79, she returns for her annual check-up again

this summer, some 21 and one-half years after her coronary occlusion.

Male — aged 58, first seen July 6, 1951.

This man had a coronary occlusion proven by electrocardiograms which showed a posterior infarction, January 10, 1951. He had always been very athletic but had had attacks of paroxysmal auricular fibrillation since he was very young. He was kept in hospital for two weeks and hadn't been able to work since six months.

He was started on 800 units of alpha tocopherol a day, and by September 18, 1951 he was "swell" — had no symptoms and was back to work. He remained well until June, 1968 (17 years!) when one evening after dinner he went out to mow the lawn. He collapsed and was taken to the hospital with auricular fibrillation. With rest and oxygen, the attack soon passed over and normal rhythm was established again. Following his release, an electrocardiogram showed no further damage, and he has been perfectly well since. He is now 76.

Male — aged 40, first seen April 8, 1949.

This man had a coronary occlusion in December, 1948, confirmed by several electrocardiograms. After recovery from the acute attack, he developed some angina on exertion.

After his being on 600 units of alpha tocopherol, these symptoms disappeared completely in four weeks. This patient, a druggist, has been perfectly well since. He owns saddle-bred, three-gaited horses and trains, rides, and shows them in the ring. He survived a severe accident with broken ribs and internal hemorrhaging in 1967 and is still active with the horses — some 20 years after his coronary occlusion.

Male — aged 51, first seen October 24, 1957.

This man was first seen after three coronary occlusions — December, 1951, 1954 and October, 1956. He had angina and dyspnea and could only walk slowly three blocks. His blood pressure and pulse were normal.

This man had no further attacks in the 12 years since we

first saw him. He very seldom has angina pectoris, has no dyspnea, lives normally, and enjoys it. He is now 63 years old.

Female — aged 56, first seen September 18, 1954.

This patient suffered a coronary occlusion in March, 1953, and her blood pressure at this time was 220 systolic. She was unable to work in her profession, that of a school teacher, until March, 1954.

After two months on 800 units of alpha tocopherol, she was able to resume her teaching, which she continued until retirement. Now, aged 71, she lives normally, has a large vegetable garden, which she tends by herself, and walks daily to the post office and back, a distance of half a mile, without distress of any kind.

Male — aged 45, April 3, 1950.

This man had a coronary occlusion in February of 1950. He was kept in bed three weeks and resting for four weeks. Apparently, some cardiologists even in 1950 were abbreviating the traditional "six weeks in bed" routine. Blood pressure and pulse rate were normal, and he was started immediately on 375 units of alpha tocopherol. Six weeks later he started back to work part time and then to full-time work as a sales executive. He was playing golf and living normally.

In 1959 he began to have a noise in the ears with some diminution of hearing, and for this reason his intake of alpha tocopherol was raised to 800 units; and 50,000 units of vitamin A were added. He remained perfectly well, except for his ear problem, which an excellent otologist considered a circulatory problem. On 1,600 units of alpha tocopherol, 50,000 units of vitamin A, and the Arlidin prescribed for him by the aforementioned otologist, there has been no deterioration in his hearing in the last ten years, but also no improvement. He can carry on his business, but must listen carefully.

He has curled (a Scottish and Canadian sport) every winter, sweeping in his turn, and plays golf regularly. He is officially retired, but working harder than ever helping a former associate to run a new firm in the same business category.

Irish woman doctor — diabetic, hypertensive, coronary thrombosis.

This woman, aged 55, cabled for an appointment from Ireland. Since her history illustrates the effect of alpha tocopherol on diabetes mellitus, angina pectoris, hypertension, and coronary thrombosis, it is worth recording in detail. The professional aspects are also worth reporting.

She was a graduate in medicine from an English university, married an Irishman, and pracficed, therefore, in Ireland. She first developed diabetes mellitus and went to England for consultation on this condition. She was hospitalized and her diabetes controlled and a regime mapped out for her. On return to Ireland she found that she could not carry on her practice on the diet prescribed, so she modified her treatment to allow her good control but enough strength to allow full-time work.

As is the rule with female diabetics, vascular changes began to occur, and she developed a moderate to severe hypertension. This was followed by angina pectoris, which gradually became more severe. After some months of angina, she suffered a severe coronary thrombosis with myocardial infarction.

After release from hospital she journeyed to the London Heart Institute for evaluation and suggested therapy. Of course, this consisted of decreased activity and nitroglycerin for angina. In spite of this, she just wasn't able to practice and retired to the country.

In her country retreat she was accompanied by one of her Great Dane dogs, a champion female. Twice this dog routed out intruders, and when the dog became older and somewhat feeble, the doctor was anxious to keep her alive and well so she sought the help of Dr. Lambert, at that time president of the Irish Veterinary Association. Dr. Lambert examined the dog, suggested treatment, but then said to the doctor, "however, I can help you a lot better than I can your dog." He prescribed a useful daily intake of vitamin E (alpha tocopherol).

The patient responded slowly to the alpha tocopherol. First, she noted a decrease in her insulin requirement, then her angina pectoris lessened and eventually disappeared, and she discovered that her blood pressure had returned to normal.

The reader, if he has read this book to this point, will realize that the doctor was unusually lucky in many ways. First of all, the dose of alpha tocopherol suggested by Dr. Lambert was exactly right. Secondly, she was one of the lucky one-third whose pressure *falls* on alpha tocopherol therapy. One-third stay at approximately the same level and one-third rise — often to tremendous heights. Thirdly, she was one of the lucky one-third of the victims of diabetes mellitus whose insulin requirement drops. Finally, her angina pectoris was completely relieved.

She returned to practice; and she felt that she could safely travel to Canada to see her elder son, his Canadian wife, and her first grandchild. She had never seen the latter two. She combined this trip with an appointment with me.

I had nothing to suggest but a continuation of the same treatment and was both interested and amused when this very professional and polite Irish woman doctor, with a delightful Irish accent, asked me two questions: the first to explain the mode of action of alpha tocopherol and then diffidently, "Why do I, who know every important doctor in England, have to be cured of my disease by my veterinarian?"

Dr. Lambert alertly picked up our original short paragraph announcement in *Nature* of our use of alpha tocopherol in cardiac disease and applied it to his veterinary practice with spectacular results, which he then published in both the *English* and *American Veterinary Journals*.

He is not the only veterinarian who has successfully treated human patients with coronary artery disease. Dr. Egan in Detroit, now unfortunately deceased, and two other veterinarians in Canada that I personally know, have more human patients in their areas than I have!

CHAPTER 3.   ANGINA PECTORIS

TYPICALLY, AN ATTACK OF ANGINA pectoris is described by the patient as a sensation of pressure, tightness, or heaviness behind the breastbone. It may become crushing in nature like a closing vise and may be very severe indeed. It can come on so suddenly that it seems instantaneous, with the victim suddenly subjected to unbearable pain that renders him unable even to walk. The attack can end quickly or can continue until it is treated. The pain has a tendency to radiate, usually to the left shoulder and arm all the way down to the fingers. It is often accompanied by great anxiety and a fear of impending death. A mild attack, however, may occur simply as a sensation of pressure within the chest.

Yet unless there is definite electrocardiographic evidence of coronary insufficiency — s-t segment and T wave changes can sometimes be elicited by taking electrocardiographic tracings immediately following or during sufficient exercise to elicit the pain — it is only by the most thorough and painstaking examination that the physician can be sure he is indeed dealing with cardiac anoxia and not with referred pain from some other disease. Since the electrocardiogram will usually show no abnormality, I have come to rely on extremely detailed case histories and an exercise trial. It is the best way I have found to distinguish true angina from its most frequent mimic, intercostal neuralgia or inflammation of one or more of the nerves between the ribs.

Characteristically, true angina pectoris is elicited when the oxygen demand is increased, which can occur because of excitement, exertion, or even after the eating of a heavy meal. However, intercostal pain may also be elicited by exertion, since an increased rate of respiration and greater movement of the chest may irritate the affected nerve, but it can also result from any change in position and frequently occurs while the patient is sitting in a chair or lying in bed, whereas true angina does not occur when the patient is at rest.

Although it had long been supposed, because angina attacks are so frequently brought on by exercise, that the syndrome resulted from insufficient oxygen supply to the heart, it was first demonstrated in 1964 when Dr. Lawrence S. Cohen of Harvard Medical School and Peter Bent Brigham Hospital found an excess of lactic acid in the heart muscle during angina attacks. Since the consistently high quantities of lactate could only have been produced in the absence of oxygen, the findings represented a remarkably clean and uncomplicated demonstration of hypoxia, as reported to the Thirteenth Annual Convention of the American College of Cardiology in New Orleans.

Since then it has gone almost unquestioned that angina is caused by oxygen lack, which knowledge should have provided the key to a treatment that would be more than palliative. The characteristics of such a treatment had become obvious. For example, it was possible for a paper in the *New England Journal of Medicine* (December 14, 1967, page 1,278) to commence with, "Because angina pectoris is a consequence of inadequate myocardial oxygenation, ideal therapy for this incapacitating symptom would be directed toward both increasing coronary blood flow and decreasing myocardial oxygen requirements."

The authors, Dr. Braunwald, Epstein, Glick, Wechsler, and Braunwald, might just as well have gone on to name alpha tocopherol as their ideal therapy if these National Heart Insitute doctors had only known it.

It has already been pointed out in the chapter on coronary occlusion that alpha tocopherol simultaneously is a powerful fibrinolytic agent, with an action that causes arterial blood clots to disintegrate, and a vasodilator that will increase the blood supply to the heart by widening the arterial lumen.

It also plays a third and equally significant role in its function, well known to food technicians everywhere, as an antioxidant.

When it is pointed out that the consumption of polyunsaturated fats reduces the serum level of vitamin E and increases the likelihood of vitamin E deficiency, that is an expression of the consequence of vitamin E's antioxidant activity. Ordinarily the essential fatty acids released into the bloodstream by polyunsaturates are highly vulnerable to peroxidation — linking their molecules one for one with molecules of oxygen. Vitamin E in the bloodstream, however, preferentially bonds with the fatty acids and prevents their oxidation. The vitamin E is destroyed in the course of this activity, which is why polyunsaturates in the diet in any quantity create a need for proportionately more of the vitamin. But by this antioxidant activity, the vitamin prevents oxygen from being converted into toxic peroxides, leaving the red cells of the blood more fully supplied with pure oxygen that the blood carries to the heart as well as all other organs.

By all these properties already existing in one drug — and that drug virtually without side effects except through overdosage in very special cases — surely this drug, alpha tocopherol, is as well tailored to be the ideal therapy for angina as any material could possibly be.

Unfortunately, alpha tocopherol remains largely unknown to the medical profession, and as a consequence the profession has wasted a frantic 20 years of search for a drug that already exists. Untold time and money have been spent in the development of amyl Nitrite, erythrityl tetranitrate, pentaerythritol Tetranitrate, and others in a long list of nitrates and nitrites, Iproniazid, and other monoamine-oxidase inhibitors. The result is usually a short-lived fad and a quick return to nitroglycerin, which has no therapeutic effect whatsoever, but is remarkably fast and effective in relieving an attack of angina.

So after years and years of search for a drug that would treat angina, the choice available to today's doctor is still whether to use the brown nitroglycerin tablets that have a chocolate base or the white tablets with a sugar base.

To the patient accustomed to walking around with a pocket full of nitroglycerin tablets and perhaps taking as many as 20 to 30 tablets a day, it could in no way represent a burden to take a few vitamin E capsules daily, thus preventing the recurrence of angina attacks in most cases, and to be able to throw away the nitroglycerin.

The complete or nearly complete prevention of angina attacks is the usual and expected result of treatment with alpha tocopherol. Angina patients are treated exactly like those who suffer the same symptoms upon recovery from a coronary occlusion. The results are comparable in every way, except that I have a vague impression that, on the whole, patients who have had a frank coronary occlusion respond somewhat better. I don't know why.

It is essential to recall that two investigators, after years of careful study of the available material and evidence, stated that in their opinion all patients who had developed angina pectoris had had a coronary occlusion, though usually of a small vessel so that the electrocardiographic changes were not diagnostic or were easily missed. If this is so, and I consider it probable, then angina represents a specific indication for preventive measures against the possibility of thrombosis.

Unless there is some contraindication, such as hypertension, an angina patient is routinely started by me on 800 international units of alpha tocopherol a day and seen at intervals of six weeks for reassessment. If no result has been obtained within six weeks, the dosage is increased by 200 to 400 international units for the next six weeks. When we reach the dose on which their symptoms are relieved, it is continued permanently.

Although the protection from a coronary thrombosis in these patients is very nearly universal, it sometimes happens that, after some years, the symptoms of angina recur. In such a case, it is necessary once again to increase the dose gradually and keep increasing it until the condition is relieved.

In discussing the successful treatment for angina, however, it must be re-emphasized that a misdiagnosis can easily be made.

There is one type of pain which is very common in middle-aged or older people which is very commonly mistaken for angina pectoris. It has been given many different names, by many different authors, although recognized as a definite entity for years. Also, the site of the responsible lesion has been identified in different locations — the sterno-costal joint, the intercostal nerve itself, or the nerve root. To make matters more confusing, it can be on either side at any level, and so the pain can be ascribed to referred pain from several different organs. The most common name for this condition is intercostal neuralgia or intercostal neuritis, and so the inference is that it is a definite lesion of the intercostal nerve. It is often referred to as a radiculitis, signifying a lesion in the nerve root. It has been called the rib syndrome. It has been often misdiagnosed as breast tumor, cholecystitis, etc.

This pain nearly always occurs in the left upper chest in front in right-handed people and in the upper right chest in front in left-handed people. In fact, this is so usually the location and so typically right or left sided, that once the patient has described it you can confidently tell him whether he is right or left handed. Characteristic of this pain is that it occurs toward the front of the chest; but it is accompanied by marked tenderness between the ribs, and this tenderness can be followed all the way around in the intercostal space right to the lateral aspects of the spine. The patient may not be aware of the tenderness until the doctor puts pressure on the area.

The author has seen hundreds of such cases, many of which have had the condition for years. There has been no very effective medical treatment available for this condition, and the author has developed his own theories and method of treatment which are very effective in nearly all — but not all — cases.

The doctor of medicine has been taught for years that minor dislocations of joints or their immobilization in an abnormal part of their range of movement cannot occur.

Therefore, the chiropractic and osteopathic approach to pain was considered necessarily based on incorrect theory and manipulation of no greater benefit than heat and massage. All this, too, has changed, and the president of the American College of Surgeons and, now, many others have attested to the value of correct manipulation in treating many joint lesions. The author has known this for 24 years. He discovered three osteopaths who could relieve chest pain of this type in most patients, often very dramatically. In one such case a man who couldn't walk 20 yards, without pain, after manipulation walked for miles up and down hill and through college grounds and climaxed it by running upstairs, where he arrived breathless and perspiring, but free of pain.

However, again by chance, a most effective medical treatment for this condition was discovered. While investigating the possible usefulness of vitamin E ointment (30 I.U. alpha tocopherol per gram of petroleum jelly), Burgess and Pritchard of the Montreal General Hospital had demonstrated its usefulness in hastening the healing of indolent ulcers and in so doing had shown that the alpha tocopherol in the ointment was absorbed by the tissues under the skin right down to the periosteum of bone. It literally walks right through the skin as if it weren't there. Now we treat all such patients by the inunction of vitamin E ointment into the skin over the nerve root for ten minutes, followed by heat for another ten minutes to drive in still more alpha tocopherol. This works miracles in one to three nights. If it doesn't work within this three-day interval, we send the patient to the osteopath – not just any osteopath, of course – and if this doesn't get the desired result, we use vitamin B, hypodermically and by mouth, but with little hope that it will be successful.

Having excluded referred pain from organs and having excluded intercostal nerve pain, presumably pain that occurs in the chest on exertion or excitement (especially after a heavy meal or soon after the oxygen reserve in the heart muscle has been used up during sleep or after exertion just before elicitation of pain) is due to coronary artery narrowing and resulting myocardial anoxia.

A word is necessary about status anginosis, a condition of nearly continuous angina pectoris even at rest. In 30,000 cases, I've never seen one. I've seen patients in such deep failure that they couldn't move about at all — but no status anginosis. Early in our London, Ontario, days a patient of my brother's, an obstetrician, was seen in consultation while in the hospital at her daughter's request. She was there because of the diagnosis of status anginosis made by the internist to whom she had been sent by her family physician. My brother elicited the typical intercostal tenderness in the appropriate segment and suggested vitamin E ointment and heat as described in this chapter. She was completely cured of her status anginosis overnight.

Like all our coronary patients, angina patients are urged to lead normal lives, as far as this is possible. We restrict them in only two ways. We ask that they don't try to show anyone how much they can lift or how fast they can run. Many patients have returned to hard manual laboring on farms and in factories without subsequent trouble.

There is even a distinct possibility that such hard work does them good — as long as they are protected against sudden insufficiency by vitamin E saturation. It was reported by Doctors Smith and Kidera in *Aerospace Medicine* (38: 742, July, 1967) that physical stress is beneficial in some cases of angina, because it helps the development of collateral circulation. A gradually extended exercise program leading up to an objective of jogging a mile in 20 minutes showed excellent results in 15 cases and poor results in six.

The poor results, of course, were in dyspnea and early congestive failure. They could have been avoided.

CHAPTER 4. ISCHEMIC HEART DISEASE

CORONARY HEART DISEASE DUE to atherosclerosis is the clinical term for the very common entity whose chief symptom is angina pectoris, which literally means "pain of the chest."

The diagnosis of coronary heart disease is based on evidence of recent or old myocardial infarction (tissue destruction in the heart) or of angina pectoris in a patient with no evidence of syphilis or disease of the heart valves. Angina pectoris can also occur in a case of syphilitic aortitis, because the disease causes narrowing of the ostea of the coronary arteries at their origins behind cusps of the aortic valve. This can cut down the blood able to get into the coronary arteries and so lead to oxygen deficiency of the heart muscle and the production of angina pectoris. In our day this is rarely seen, however.

Angina pectoris, as we know it today, can occur with aortic stenosis, or narrowing of the aorta, and less frequently also with aortic regurgitation. Also angina pectoris does occur less frequently with mitral stenosis and congestive heart disease of noncoronary origin.

However, a definitive diagnosis of Coronary Heart Disease depends upon an unequivocal history of distinctive cardiac pain or of electrocardiographic changes denoting acute or healed myocardial infarction. Occasionally, but not often there are other manifestations that might suggest coronary heart disease, such as acute pulmonary edema, chronic congestive heart failure, systematic arterial embolization, or the onset of the Stokes-Adams syndrome. Angina remains the primary symptom.

It is necessary to point out that when patients first develop the disease, there are usually no physical signs of the condition and that the electrocardiogram is ordinarily normal.

Angina occurs when the lumen of the artery is diminished to about one-third of its normal size, either in a small area or in a more diffuse change. The pain is typically behind the breastbone (sternum) or across the chest. It is commonly described as a tight band across the chest or like a heavy weight over the sternum. It may be referred to either shoulder, though usually the left, and may extend down into the hand on the little finger side. The pain may extend into the jaw or teeth instead of into the shoulder or arm region. The symptom is brought on by exertion, usually walking outdoors, by emotion, commonly after ingestion of a heavy meal, by tachycardia in the susceptible, and by cold, especially by walking in the cold.

Angina, as a symptom following coronary occlusion, has been fully discussed in the chapter dealing with that subject. What we are dealing with now is a condition with no clinical or electrocardiographic signs. However, there is a general acceptance of the definitive work of Blumgart and Schlesinger, who showed that at autopsy the hearts of subjects who had suffered angina during life contained at least one and usually two scars of previous coronary occlusions.

Present statistics indicate that the average length of life after the onset of angina pectoris is about ten years and that myocardial infarction or congestive heart failure are the usual causes of death in such patients.

One of the curious situations that we are faced with time after time is the frank delight of the patient who has been very ill with heart disease and who has had a complete return to apparently normal health. His secondary reaction so often is a bewildered question: "Why have the doctors not generally adopted this treatment?" Some of these patients have become very belligerent and are hard to calm down, since they consider their own physicians have let them suffer needlessly and, callously and unconcernedly, let them proceed toward death.

We are unable to help them in this phase, since there are organizations, notably Heart Associations, which raise large sums of money and profess to be fighting heart disease. Yet they have done as near to nothing as is possible while feeding large sums of money into research institutions, which promptly spend it with absolutely no results whatsoever. To make matters worse, a large number of leading cardiologists, including the man whose name is currently most famous, *know* that vitamin E is at least a partial answer. Why they have done nothing but ignore or oppose it must be because it is still not politically wise.

The same situation occurs when anyone, such as an author or a drug salesman, is introduced to vitamin E and sees what it can do medically. He is originally uninterested, then becomes curious, and soon becomes an angry evangelist. To us, who have gone through this for more than 20 years, this stage has mercifully passed, and we go about our business of helping as many patients as we can who find their way to us.

However, there is a time and place for everything, and the time has come when it should be pointed out that the average cardiologist can do nothing to help a damaged heart if *he does not use vitamin E* — except to treat symptoms and complications.

Let the cardiologist tell you about it himself. For this we quote the editorial in the *Texas State Journal of Medicine* of January, 1951, written by George W. Parson, M.D., president of the Texas State Heart Association.

The Challenge of Cardiovascular Disease

More than 637,000 deaths annually in the United States from cardiovascular disease account for about 44 per cent of all deaths. Approximately 9,000,000 Americans have heart disease; of these 500,000 are elementary and high school children. An estimated 152,100,000 workdays are lost each year because of diseases of the heart and blood vessels. This is the challenge of cardiovascular disease.

Equally as challenging is the individual patient. When a physician makes a diagnosis of organic heart disease, he realizes that in the care of the patient he has begun a losing fight. In the earliest stages he offers general advice; "avoid strenuous activities; live sensibly; watch your weight; don't worry; the heart is a wonderful organ." Before long symptoms develop and the doctor braces the patient with digitalis or other drugs, restriction of usual activities, more rest and more encouragement. Again, before long, more urgent symptoms force a retreat. Bedrest, low sodium diet, diuretics, and other well known measures are brought to the front and the line is stabilized. But not for long. All too soon increasing pressure bends the line and retreat begins again. Now there are left no more reserves — no more in the heart and no more in the hands of the one trying to help the heart. Then only surrender remains. Not infrequently the enemy strikes suddenly with overwhelming power, and surrender occurs before the doctor can mobilize his forces.

This is not to minimize our present efforts. Our forces are better trained and more efficient than they ever have been, and we are able to hold the line longer than ever before. But present day efforts are not enough. Much more education and research will be needed before the course of cardiovascular disease can be reversed or its development prevented. The control of heart disease is a great challenge to every physician and layman."

George W. Parson, M.D., President
Texas Heart Association,
Texas State Journal of Medicine,
January, 1951.

This editorial could just as well have been written in January, 1969, since it is just as true today as it was in 1951.

I have before me a pamphlet sent out by the Florida Heart Association, a member of the American Heart Association, and I cannot think of any more pitiful literature. It certainly must depress the recipient if he reads carefully. For the sufferer from angina pectoris, it states, "Most angina patients can look forward to years of active living." Reducing activity, working at a less demanding job, getting lots of rest, and the use of nitroglycerin is all there is to suggest. How could there be less?

Meanwhile, it has been established by many workers that alpha tocopherol decreases the need of oxygen in heart muscle and that it reduces the tendency to thrombosis. What more does one need than that and the published successes of hundreds of internists, surgeons, biochemists, veterinarians, etc., throughout the civilized world?

One of my patients had the answer! He was the largest exporter of day-old chicks by plane to Japan and told me a parallel story of his experience. The Canadian Poultry Association holds an annual convention at which there is always a featured guest speaker, followed by open and usually rather frank discussion. Some years ago, the guest speaker came from California and outlined a completely new and very radical method of raising chicks for the commercial market. It was so new as to appear, on the face of it, quite ridiculous. He was "taken apart" by the audience, and two professors from the poultry department of our Agricultural College were most critical and advised the assembled members to have nothing to do with it, giving very logical and scientific reasons for their stand. The Californian chicken farmer kept cool and reasonable, answered their questions, but kept repeating: "Gentlemen, why don't you try it? It works." Then my patient told me, "You know every successful chicken farmer in Canada is now using this method and do you know who are teaching it to the upcoming poultry farmers? Those two professors from the agricultural school." Then he said, "Dr. Shute, you should never say anything about vitamin E, except 'Why don't you try it? It works.'"

Of course, like every other potent medication, it doesn't work for everyone. The wide variation in its oxygen-sparing activity in different patients means that some get absolute relief as long as they take the optimum dosage while others get nearly complete relief. Some get definite help but still need occasional nitroglycerin.

I have mentioned elsewhere, I believe, that we have had as patients three of the richest men in Canada and England. I do so only because they are obviously in a position to obtain the services of the best-known cardiologists in England, Canada, or the U.S. There must be a reason why they chose us. One of these cases will illustrate the point.

This man, his whole family, and the chief executive of virtually each one of his numerous world-wide companies are all patients as a result of the coronary occlusion suffered by his mother-in-law.

She was at his northern Ontario camp some 50 miles north of my own. The local doctor was called to treat her. He, in turn, summoned a cardiologist from the nearest city, who in turn sent for a cardiologist from our leading Canadian university. All three, after consultation, informed the family that she had had a very extensive myocardial infarction, that she could not be moved, and that she would certainly die and that very soon. After they left, the son-in-law called the Shute Institute in London to ask if there was any help available and was told where he might locate me, since I was in the immediate area. He failed to reach me, but three days later when I was on my way home, I was intercepted at the next village and asked to call the northern lodge.

The patient's granddaughter, along with special nurses, was looking after the patient and was able to give me all the necessary data about her case, her blood pressure, her pulse rate, whether it showed normal sinus rhythm, or not (it did), as well as the presence or absence of congestive failure, orthopnea, dsypnea, etc. I suggested the routine we used in such patients to the daughter, who dutifully copied it down. Then, the son-in-law returned to the phone and asked me what I thought and how she would respond. He wanted to know when she could be moved, since her home was in one of the Southern states, some 1,500 miles or more away. I told him she would be better on the tenth day, could sit up out of bed in three weeks, and go south in six.

She was better on the tenth day, sat out of bed after three weeks, and went to Virginia after six weeks, perfectly well.

This man said that if I could tell him she would live, could tell him the exact day she would be well, the exact day she could get out of bed, and the exact day she could safely travel, he had better come over to our side.

Any physician reading this can do as well, since this was about the third year of my experience with vitamin E, some 17 or 18 summers ago.

A few case histories follow:

Male — aged 52, seen first September 24, 1968.

This man developed angina in March of 1968. It would begin substernally and, if it continued for any length of time, extend upward into his neck. Nitroglycerin relieved this pain. He made an appointment because the attacks were becoming more severe and more prolonged. Shortness of breath usually accompanied the pain, but might disappear just before the pain began. Palpitation usually accompanied both the pain and the dyspnea. He was able to walk two blocks to the post office, but developed the pain on returning, since it was a little "up grade." His blood pressure was 110/70, pulse 52.

On 1,200 units of alpha tocopherol, his angina disappeared entirely by the fourth week of treatment. Now, five months later, he has been walking regularly about two miles a day and is now jogging a little with no distress. His blood pressure is 120/70, pulse 56.

Female — aged 47 when first seen November 4, 1949.

This woman had developed angina pectoris slowly over the course of the previous two years. At this time we were using approximately 300 units of alpha tocopherol a day, and on this dosage she developed severe congestive failure and needed mercurial diuretics. It wasn't until October, 1952, when her dosage was raised to 375 units that her angina disappeared and her failure came under control.

By May, 1953, she stated that "she was feeling so well, working like a hatter." She had no pain and no dyspnea, and all her peripheral edema was gone.

In the intervening years, with much family illness and

one or two broken bones, she has had several brief episodes of peripheral edema and a little congestive failure, but has carried on a perfectly normal life with perhaps more activity than most people.

She is now 67. For the last month she has been confined to a nursing home after a fall April 17, 1969, in which she sustained a broken hip and right arm!

Male.

This man volunteered for the army in 1943, at the age of 37, as a commando. As the training period in Canada neared its end and just before they were scheduled to go overseas, he developed on exertion pain in the very center of his chest. Eventually, during one of the final route marches, he was unable to continue after three miles and dropped out. He was very embarrassed by his distress and by its timing and only reported it when, on this occasion, he could not carry on. He succeeded in getting the final decision on his status with the unit deferred — until, while on leave, he was able to obtain a careful examination by one of the senior Canadian cardiologists. He confirmed the diagnosis of coronary insufficiency, with angina pectoris, and stated that he couldn't possibly continue in army service.

He consulted me on March 13, 1947, and since blood pressure, pulse, and resting electrocardiogram were normal, was started on 400 units daily of alpha tocopherol. Ten days later, he felt definite improvement, and recovery was nearly complete between the third and fourth weeks of treatment and complete by the sixth week.

He has been called up annually by the medical board of the Veterans' Hospital and is usually questioned at length about his treatment with vitamin E. On one occasion, just to test the reaction of his examining physician, he stated that he had stopped this treatment. The physician became fairly agitated, walked up and down for awhile, and finally said, "You're the biggest damn fool I've seen today. You know what it has done for you, why did you stop it?" He then went on to say he wasn't *allowed* to prescribe it in the Department of Veterans' Affairs, but "it certainly was good."

Ischemic Heart Disease

This man's first symptoms began at age 37. He is now 64, works every day, and lives a normal life. He has just survived an episode of pneumonia following an attack of the "Hong Kong flu," a severe test of his cardiac condition.

He has had 27 years of normal health following the onset of severe coronary insufficiency, severe enough to invalid him out of the army on an army pension. Our army doesn't pay pensions on "suspected" coronary disease!

Here is the history of a man who retired twice, years apart, on pension.

This man came to us first on June 16, 1952, at the age of 48. He had severe angina pectoris on exertion and was off work.

On alpha tocopherol he was free of pain by November 1, 1952, but was retired from his job as a railroad section foreman on a pension of $50.00 a month.

On vitamin E, he was returned to "good health" with very rare brief attacks of angina pectoris.

He went back to work at a new job and has just been retired on a second pension at age 65 (compulsory retirement age).

CHAPTER 5. RHEUMATIC FEVER and ACUTE RHEUMATIC HEART DISEASE

ALTHOUGH ACUTE RHEUMATIC fever is a distressing and sometimes fatal illness, usually with a variety of painful symptoms, it is the frequency with which it leads to rheumatic heart disease that, above all other considerations, demands rapid and effective treatment. Rheumatic heart disease, in turn, is the commonest form of heart disease in children and is responsible for 90 per cent of defective hearts among the young.

It is also the second most prevalent form of heart disease in adults, accounting for 30 per cent of crippled hearts and about 50 per cent of the deaths from heart disease that occur before 30 years of age. It is the cause of death of between 30,000 and 60,000 people in the U.S. yearly.

The average life of patients with definitive rheumatic heart disease is about 15 years after its onset. About 50 per cent live less than nine years. In adults, about 75 per cent of sufferers from rheumatic heart disease die as a direct result, mostly due to congestive heart failure, while about 10 per cent die of thrombosis or infarction, and about six per cent develop bacterial endocarditis, inflammation of membranous and connective tissues of the heart. Clearly the responsible rheumatic fever is a major medical problem.

Rheumatic fever is not a "reportable" disease, and so there are no accurate statistics available for many of its aspects. It is known that most cases are preceded by a few weeks, usually about three, by an acute infection with hemolytic streptococci group A, usually type 12, in the nose, paranasal sinuses, pharynx, pharyngeal lymphatic tissue, or tonsils. The mortality from the acute attack averages one to four per cent but nearly 85 per cent of those with rheumatic fever develop rheumatic heart disease. Rheumatic heart disease is now generally recognized as a chronic infection.

There are many curious features of this disease worth mentioning here. First of all, there are no specific diagnostic features, and the patient or his family may not be aware that he is ill. On the other hand, he may have evidence of involvement of the serous (serum-producing) membranes of joints or those enveloping the brain and spinal cord of pleura or pericardium and be acutely ill with all gradations in between these two states. Involuntary jerky movements (chorea) and circular reddened areas on the skin, with elevated edges, are other important diagnostic signs. Daily or semiweekly electrocardiograms shows transitory abnormalities in more than 95 per cent of hospitalized patients, which suggests that most victims of rheumatic fever have heart damage.

As a result of the great variation in the initial symptoms and the lack of specific diagnostic criteria, the patient with rheumatic heart disease may be totally unaware of his condition, until he develops progressive breathlessness on exertion or an attack of acute shortness of breath or the gradual appearance of peripheral edema, several years later.

Although a specific group A hemolytic streptococcal infection precedes the rheumatic fever, treatment of the latter by the sulfonamides or penicillin is useless. Yet, the gradual decrease in the incidence of rheumatic heart disease is almost certainly due to the adequate treatment with these drugs of patients with the preceding streptococcal infection. In a word, rheumatic heart disease can be prevented by antibiotic therapy, but not treated.

The reason that this subject is so important and that this chapter follows after the chapters on coronary artery disease, is that there is a most successful treatment for the acute and early stages of rheumatic heart disease. On the other hand, there is no evidence that any of the currently popular forms of treatment has any effect upon the progress of the disease. Rest in bed, suppression of pain and fever, etc., while making the patient more comfortable do not alter the damage to the structures or to the progress of the disease.

Currently, the disease is usually regarded as an allergic phenomenon since it has been shown that the poison affects the whole of the cardiovascular tree with the most serious damage affecting the heart muscles and the valves of the heart. The pathologists have described a typical lesion as affecting the "ground substance" of the connective tissue, although Murphy has shown that the Aschoff nodule may result from rheumatic injury to the heart muscle cell with its eventual disintegration and replacement with scar tissue.

The initial damage done by rheumatic fever occurs in the region surrounding the blood vessels that supply the heart muscle and the serum-producing membranes. In the heart the perivascular reaction causes areas of injury with fluid accumulation and the collection of inflammatory cells. Small areas of myocardium — heart muscle — are destroyed, and the final result is a myocardium full of many, many small areas of scar tissue. The inflammation of the serous membranes lining the heart, inside and out, leads to injury, scarring, and eventually scar-tissue contraction. Since the valves are folds of endocardium, they become involved in 85 per cent of cases. The scarring and contraction lead to thickening and narrowing of the valves, with a decrease in the size of the orifice when the valve is open, or it may be so distorted as to be unable to close completely, or both.

These lesions attack the valves directly at the line of opposition of the opposing cusps, with thickening of the valve, eventual scarring and deformity, and shortening of the chordae tendinae.

With good recovery from the acute attack of rheumatic fever, with an average degree of damage to the heart muscle and valves, there is usually a quiescent period during which the patient may be apparently perfectly well. Indeed, such a person may engage in vigorous athletics successfully for years without knowing he has heart damage. In my own experience, professional football and baseball athletes and Olympic skating and swimming competitors are numbered among my rheumatic heart disease cripples.

To summarize:

Rheumatic fever is a vicious disease, sometimes difficult to diagnose in its early stages, sometimes escaping detection during its acute phase. Whenever it attacks a patient, there is usually some damage to the heart, and no treatment currently used, except the alpha tocopherol treatment about to be described, has been shown to do anything to alter its inexorable course.

Apart from the one to four per cent, who die in the acute stage, it is a chronic disease, with progessive damage to heart valves and heart muscle, leading to recurrences of the acute phase or to the final stages of chronic rheumatic heart disease.

The actions of alpha tocopherol which affect the acute rheumatic fever and the early stages of the cardiac complications, or the similar state in a recurrent attack of rheumatic fever, are those which diminish the allergic reactions in the cardiovascular tree, those that prevent capillary thrombosis and consequent tissue destruction, and those which decrease the oxygen need of the tissue.

Alpha tocopherol's ability to return abnormal capillaries to normal reduces fluid accumulation within and between cells, promotes normal gas interchange across the involved cell membranes, and seems thereby to halt the disease very rapidly. Decreased oxygen need allows rapid recovery and rapid healing.

The effect of alpha tocopherol in acute rheumatic fever can best be illustrated by two cases, the first one ever so treated and a more recent one.

Twenty-three years ago, I was called out to a neighboring farm to see an acutely ill boy of 15 years. When 11 years old, the lad had had an attack of acute rheumatic fever and was treated in the most famous Canadian hospital for sick children, where he was kept for seven months on the ward and was then sent to that hospital's convalescent hospital, where he remained a patient for another 15 months before returning home to his family's farm. After some weeks at home, he was permitted to do minor chores that were not physically taxing, such as feeding the chickens. He gradually increased his activity until the summer of 1946, when, while riding the tractor, he developed pain in one wrist and, within 24 hours, had a definite migrating acute rheumatic fever.

When I examined him, his temperature was 100.3, his pulse 120, and three joints were involved. The wrist which had been acutely involved was by now almost normal again; one knee was acutely inflamed and swollen, and the other knee was beginning to be involved. The tags remaining from a tonsillectomy, which had been performed while he was in the original hospital, had become reddened and inflamed.

His heart was moderately enlarged and showed the typical murmurs of mitral stenosis — narrowing of the orifice on the left side of the heart — and of mitral regurgitation, due to incomplete closure of the valve.

The only treatment I used for the boy was 200 units of alpha tocopherol daily. In three days he was apparently well, and on the sixth day he walked into my office. He was able to return to normal farm activities.

In November of that same year, 1946, along with several other of my patients, he was examined by four eminent university staff cardiologists, who remarked on the existing cardiac enlargement and the murmurs. When they questioned him about his physical condition, however, he told them that he had just spent four days pulling turnips.

Since then, he has remained perfectly well; has grown into a tall, well-developed man; has done all sorts of manual labor, including one summer's work harvesting grain in the Canadian west, and since then has worked in a feed mill where the labor is taxing.

When I was first called to see this boy, his mother remarked that she didn't know how she could face another 22 months of hospitalization and subsequent convalescence. He was the thirteenth child in the family, and obviously his mother had her hands full with her entire brood. I could offer no reassurance at that time, for this was the first case in all the world in which rheumatic fever had been treated with vitamin E. Fortunately the result obtained exceeded even my hopes. His total convalescence was six days.

One day in July, 1968, a 20-year-old neighbor, who had just finished his first year in pharmacy and who was working for the summer in the service department of a large tire manufacturing company, developed soreness of his left wrist. This was on a Friday morning. The company doctor put the joint at rest with a palmar splint, and by the following Monday the wrist was nearly pain-free, and he returned to work. Monday afternoon he developed a sore, swollen left knee, and the company doctor diagnosed acute rheumatic fever and sent him home to his family physician. Since he was the son of the patient described in the chapter on acute coronary occlusion, his mother phoned me. I had her take him to the hospital laboratory for sedimentation rate, white blood cell count, etc., and after my afternoon office hours called on him at home. By this time his right knee was swollen and sore, he was running a fever, and was willing to admit he was in real pain. He was started immediately on 800 I.U. of alpha tocopherol and was perfectly well 48 hours later — clinically and by all known laboratory tests.

On the third day, Thursday, I surprised him, up and dressed and entertaining two of his college chums, who were trying to throw him into their back yard swimming pool. He was successfully resisting them when I came by.

By any other method of treatment, he would, of necessity, have been weeks or months in bed, his pain controlled by aspirin, salicylates, or cortisone, but his basic condition not one whit helped. His future might well have been altered materially since 85 per cent of such patients develop permanent cardiac damage.

Now, one year later, he is apparently perfectly well, and there is no detectable evidence of any cardiac damage.

Still another early case, a boy of 12 years seen in the children's hospital in consultation, illustrates the rapid recovery possible with alpha tocopherol and no other treatment. This lad had a typical acute rheumatic fever with evidence of severe cardiac involvement. It was when the family physician, and the specialist he had called in, explained the seriousness of the condition and the grave prognosis that the father asked that I be called in as a consultant. He had developed pericardial and pleural effusion in addition to his joint involvement.

At the time he was seen, we were cautiously using larger doses of the drug and started him on 600 units a day. His symptoms disappeared by the third day, his pericardial and pleural effusions completely by the sixth day. He was discharged from the hospital on the tenth day and has remained perfectly well since — a matter of 19 years or so.

Two of our earliest cases of acute rheumatic fever have interesting stories worth recounting. One, first seen in 1948 during an acute recurrence of the disease and with the characteristic murmurs of mitral stenosis, did characteristically well with alpha tocopherol treatment. In 1954, he had joined the Royal Canadian Air Force. Although he had told them his cardiac history, exhaustive examination revealed no evidence of the disease. On his first leave he came to me for a check-up, and I was also unable to find any evidence of rheumatic heart disease.

The second case is similar in all respects, except that he applied for enrollment in a forestry survey camp in northern Ontario. Here also the well-established murmurs, typical of rheumatic heart disease with mitral stenosis, had disappeared.

I was fortunate enough to examine a Royal Canadian Air Force veteran, who had been discharged from the service almost exactly two years after an initial attack of rheumatic fever. On his discharge, careful examination had revealed no murmur. Three months later I examined him for entrance into the local agricultural college under the Department of Veterans' Affairs. At this time, he had a definite presystolic mitral murmur, although he felt perfectly well. With alpha tocopherol, it gradually lessened and had disappeared by the fourth month. When last seen, six years later, there was no evidence of heart damage.

We, of course, have many such patients who have lived normal lives and remained well after adequate treatment in childhood of acute or recurrent acute rheumatic fever, and the response of patients seen more recently has been the same.

For example, one first seen May 29, 1967, at the age of nine years, will illustrate the point. He was interesting, because he was the only child of an unusual couple. The father was Japanese, a black belt jujitsu expert and teacher and the mother a white Caucasian, apt pupil of the art.

The lad had an attack of acute rheumatic fever in January, 1963 and has since had a recurrent fever of 101 to 102.3 with any exertion. He suffered from epistaxis once or twice a week and perspired excessively with the slightest exertion. He was markedly short of breath on exertion. Following his attack of acute rheumatic fever, when symptoms did not subside, he was kept in bed from September, 1964 until December, 1965. He continued to show fever all the while. From December, 1965 to April of 1966 he was partially confined to bed, since he had to learn to walk all over again. His mother then took him to California for two months where she heard about vitamin E treatment, and she started to give him 50 to 100 units daily. His temperature fell to normal for the most part, and his general condition started to improve.

I accidentally met his mother who was standing beside a friend of mine in a large crowd at a dog show, the friend talking about my use of vitamin E. However, the boy did not come to me for examination or treatment for some months.

On examination, there was nothing remarkable except for a faint presystolic murmur at the apex. His temperature was normal when seen in the office. I raised his dose of alpha tocopherol to 300 units a day, and he improved steadily over the next six weeks. He has been playing ball, without distress or fever, and he has remained clinically well since.

A 16-year-old girl, first seen on October 31, 1967, had not been well since an infection in April of 1967, the condition complicated by an allergy to grasses. She did not respond to antibiotics and in spite of treatment, developed severe pains in her left chest. X-rays showed a pleural effusion, treated by a change in antibiotics, but she was not told to go to bed. She became very tired, ran a chronic fever, and when she tried to run became dyspneic and cyanotic, a condition of insufficient oxygenation characterized by blueness of the skin. Her mother took her to the Cleveland Clinic at the end of August, 1967, and after exhaustive laboratory X-ray and other tests, she was diagnosed as having mitral regurgitation. She was given penicillin and released from the clinic. She showed no improvement up to the time she presented herself to me on October 31, 1967.

Her heart was well "up to size," her blood pressure 100/40. She was cyanotic, and she showed a definite mitral regurgitation. She was started immediately on 300 units of alpha tocopherol daily. By December 13, 1967, she was "fine," ever so much better, free of fever, and had very little, if any, cyanosis. By February, 1968, she was active in sports with no handicaps and could swim without dyspnea.

Except for acute thrombophlebitis and acute glomerulonephritis, there is nothing so dramatic in this field of medicine as the response to adequate vitamin E therapy in acute rheumatic fever.

CHAPTER 6. *CHRONIC RHEUMATIC HEART DISEASE*

AS PREVIOUSLY STATED, THIS IS the second most common form of heart disease and accounts for 30 per cent of the crippled hearts in the adult. It is the cause of death in 30,000 to 60,000 persons annually in the U.S. It accounts for virtually all heart disease deaths between the ages of five and 25 years—50 per cent of all deaths before the age of 30.

There had been no treatment available to prevent the onset of this disease until the sulfonamide and antibiotic era. However, since the general use of these drugs, the incidence of rheumatic fever and, consequently, of rheumatic heart disease, has been decreasing. This is because adequate treatment of invasion of the body by group A hemolytic streptococci, usually type 12, and its elimination prevent the allergic response of the body, some three weeks or so later, that is rheumatic fever.

Unfortunately, in this context, many doctors use the sulfonamides and penicillin as infrequently as possible, no doubt due to the emphasis that was put on the dangers of their use when first introduced, but also because of the definite evidence now that their indiscriminate use and misuse have led to the development of resistant strains of virulent streptococci and staphylococci for which no antibiotic is effective.

Consequently, many children are not treated by antibiotics for their streptococcal infections, either because they are not presented to the doctor or the doctor elects not to use an antibiotic.

Of course, there are still those individuals who had their acute attacks of rheumatic fever before the antibiotic era and so are today suffering from chronic rheumatic heart disease. Again, no accurate statistics are available, but it is believed that one to six per cent of the general population have specific rheumatic valvular defects.

These valvular defects consist of scarring of the cusps and shortening of the chordae tendinae. The resulting loss of efficiency in the functioning of the heart valves often leads to regurgitation—the backward flow of blood that has already passed through the valve in the correct forward direction. The most commonly involved valve is the mitral — the only one of the four that has but two cusps, which may account for its increased susceptibility.

The aortic valve is also commonly affected, while the pulmonic valve is rarely deformed, and the tricuspid valve also usually escapes deformity. Narrowing of the mitral valve is more common than mitral regurgitation and the combination is more common than either alone. On the other hand, aortic regurgitation is five times more common than aortic stenosis. Both aortic stenosis (narrowing of the aorta) and regurgitation are often combined, and rarely is there aortic stenosis alone.

A recent discussion of chronic rheumatic heart disease in the *British Medical Journal* (May, 1968) points out the grave characteristics of the disease and, better than any recent article, implies the total lack of any accepted treatment for the condition except surgery. In fact, the author advocates surgical treatment "as soon as it is certain that the valvular defect is of serious hemodynamic significance; that is to say the degree of stenosis or incompetence is causing objective evidence of severity *whether or not symptoms are present.*" The italics are the author's, not mine.

He stresses the fact that when the surgeons found they could open the heart they found that, more often than not, the medical diagnosis and assessment of the pathological processes present were quite wrong.

The author's reason for advocating early surgery is the established fact that the disease is chronic and that it leads to progressive changes in the pulmonary circulation in the right ventricle and also, if there is cardiac failure, in the lungs.

The author admits the obvious fact that surgery does not halt the rheumatic process and that the progressive sclerosis and calcification of the valve continues.

We have seen many hundreds of such cases over the last 20-odd years and while it is the hardest of all the various types of heart disease to treat, it is the most satisfactory in the long run. Virtually all those with early symptoms and normal sinus rhythm respond well and continue to improve slowly for many months. The more advanced cases are, in many instances, very difficult to treat, and require patient, careful attention for many weeks, initially. Yet, some of our most advanced cases have shown unexpected magnificent improvement.

I have, of course, also followed with extreme interest the course of surgical treatment of these patients in many cardiac centers, since I have not wanted to be responsible for withholding help, directly or indirectly, from any patients by the use of an inferior form of treatment. Also, I have been fortunate in having had as a clinical instructor in medical school the most brilliant surgeon Canada has ever produced. He was one of the first, perhaps the first, to attempt correction of mitral stenosis surgically. The last time I talked to him, he said he was going to abandon surgery of the rheumatic heart until it was obvious that the long-term result was worthwhile.

While hoping that improved surgical methods may make surgery superior to alpha tocopherol, at the time of writing it is obvious that alpha tocopherol is by far the best form of treatment available to the sufferer from chronic rheumatic heart disease. Certainly the type of patient that Dr. Turner suggests should be submitted to surgery will do very well indeed with alpha tocopherol therapy and will never need surgery. The far advanced case will do better with alpha tocopherol as well.

It seems very hard to me to evaluate the results of surgical treatment in a patient "whether or not symptoms are present." On the other hand, all the patients we see have developed symptoms, and these we remove in virtually all the early cases.

There are very special characteristics of alpha tocopherol treatment in the case of the rheumatic heart disease patient, and I want to point out at the onset that the improper use of the drug may well kill the patient, while too small a dosage will have no effect whatsoever.

In general, the dosage schedule of alpha tocopherol is totally different from that used in the other forms of heart disease. Referring back to the early part of this chapter it will be obvious that in most cases the damage to the heart is more severe on one side, usually the left, than it is on the other. This is because the mitral valve, between the left auricle and the left ventricle, is the valve that is most usually affected, while the valves in the right side may be totally unaffected. In other cases, there is damage in the valve or valves as well as the myocardium on both sides and as a result the hemodynamic effect may be nearly equal.

The heart is really two organs joined together by a common central septum. The right side has less work to do than the left in that, simply stated, it takes blood brought to it by the great veins and propels it into the pulmonary tree. On the other hand, the left side takes blood from the lungs and sends it around miles of steadily narrowing blood vessels. Consequently, the muscular wall of the left ventricle is much thicker than that of the right ventricle. When one side of the heart is unable to keep up its work normally because of abnormalities of the valves, while the other side is functioning well, fluid collects in the tissues proximal to the malfunctioning side, and the two sides of the heart are "out of balance." Give such a patient a large dose of alpha tocopherol, and the good side improves faster than the poor side, the imbalance is increased, and the congestive failure becomes rapidly worsened. Continuation of large daily doses of alpha tocopherol will lead to rapid worsening and, if not withdrawn, to the patient's death.

The object of treatment, therefore, is to help the more damaged side of the heart very gradually and to bring its efficiency up so slowly that it comes into normal balance with that of the good side. Then when the effective dose level is reached, the heart acting as a single unit will begin to improve.

Again, let me emphasize this unique response of the chronic rheumatic heart when treatment with alpha tocopherol is instituted.

Since we are unable to predict which patients can tolerate a fair-sized initial dose, a slow, cautious routine is now invariably used. It nearly always leads to eventual worthwhile improvement in such cases. We tell all such patients now that they can expect improvement to a worthwhile degree in approximately three to three and one-half months but will see none at all short of that length of time. If their condition is progressively worsening, it will continue to do so for the first three months or so, and they must use all the help available in the meantime from decreased activity, digitalis, or even diuretics, if needed, to control the symptoms of their disease. If the patient responds as expected, there will be no doubt in his mind or his physicians' that he is definitely improved. He can be confidently advised that his condition will continue to improve slowly but steadily for many months.

Precise Dosage Is Crucial To Avoid Deterioration

In a few cases, after about eight weeks there is a definite improvement, then a worsening. This is evidence that even the dosage schedule is "too much, too soon," so the alpha tocopherol should be stopped for a day and a half, recommenced at a slightly lower dosage level, and increased more slowly.

This dosage schedule is as follows:

For the first four weeks, the patient takes 90 units a day; for the second four weeks, 120 units a day, and then 150 units a day. One hundred and fifty units is usually the maximum tolerated for many months and ordinarily is enough. If more is given and the patient is unable to tolerate it, there will be no change for seven to ten days, a little worsening around the fourteenth day, and a rapid return of unwanted symptoms thereafter. On the other hand, a dose that can be tolerated, with no change or with improvement for six weeks, will not cause regression of the cardiac status.

The ideal dosage for patients with rheumatic heart disease is 300 units a day if and when they can tolerate it. On 300 units a day, nothing untoward can happen to the patient. He is no longer a case for worry or concern.

However, most patients cannot and need not be raised to this level. It is a matter for precise medical judgment and skill. However, the characteristic of alpha tocopherol therapy so important to remember in all cases is nowhere better exemplified than in these cases. If the dose is too large, the patient will show no change for seven to ten days and will gradually worsen thereafter. Deterioration, though, will be at a sufficiently slow rate so that the doctor can take his time and check carefully to make sure that the patient really is deteriorating. When it is confirmed, stopping the use of the drug will lead to its rapid excretion and a quick drop in the level, so that no real harm is done.

This is a basic concept in alpha tocopherol treatment—the right dose of alpha tocopherol takes five to ten days to begin to act and four to six weeks before it becomes obviously effective. When the drug is stopped, it disappears from the body nearly completely after three days. Therefore, when evaluating the condition of a patient, it is necessary to remember that his present status is due to the dosage he has been taking continuously for the last month or more, not to that which he has been taking for the last week. The above applies in cardiac cases and in most peripheral vascular cases with arterial damage. In contrast, as stated elsewhere, the effects of the drug appear in hours in the patient with acute rheumatic fever, fresh thrombophlebitis or very early glomerulorphritis.

The history of my absolutely favorite patient will illustrate these principles very well. As a child, she contracted diphtheria with some weeks of soft palate paralysis, followed by rheumatic fever within weeks. She apparently made a normal recovery from these conditions except for a slight residual effect of soft palate paralysis from the diphtheria. A few years later she had scarlet fever. Her recovery was apparently complete, since when 16 years old and again when 20, she represented Canada at the Olympic Games. She was the first Canadian swimmer to break an Olympic and an American record in her specialty, the breast stroke, and was also an all-round swimmer and winner of the Gail Trophy for Ornamental Swimming.

Nevertheless, she had sustained an important degree of cardiac damage, which showed up for the first time during her second pregnancy. She was on a small dose of vitamin E to maintain this pregnancy, and an increased dose solved the problem of her congestive failure. Without our knowledge, she was treated perfectly for her cardiac condition during her two pregnancies, both of which were initiated and maintained with great difficulty by vitamin E. However, after delivery, vitamin E was deemed unnecessary, was withdrawn, and again congestive failure ensued.

On 150 units of alpha tocopherol, which was the dosage used during the last months of the second pregnancy, her congestive failure disappeared, and she was rapidly returned to apparently normal health.

Complications of Increased Dosage

By persistence, by trial and error really, her dosage was gradually increased as she was able to tolerate it. Many times it was necessary to stop for one and one half days and decrease it to the former level. It took nearly ten years before she could tolerate 300 units a day, but on this quantity she has been very well, swims, plays golf, and looks after all her own housework.

Four years ago, because she was in her mid-fifties and needed protection if possible against the danger, however remote, of a coronary thrombosis, I raised her dose of alpha tocopherol from 300 units to 375 units a day. This precipitated congestive failure with marked trouble in breathing (dyspnea), inability to get her breath lying down (orthopnea), and a cough due to fluid in the alveoli of her lung. Correction of the dosage level by stopping it for one and a half days and resumption of 300 units led to rapid and complete recovery. After nearly 19 years of alpha tocopherol and nine years of 300 units, raising her dosage from 300 to 375 units could well have been fatal.

The following cases are chosen because they were among the very first treated 23 years ago. All are still living and doing well. Obviously, they would all be dead by now but for alpha tocopherol.

The first one was seen by a group of Canadian cardiologists who commented on the gross enlargement of his heart and obvious valvular murmurs.

He gave no history of rheumatic fever and had always been healthy and rugged, enjoying outdoor activities. He was, therefore, surprised when he was rejected for army service because of evidence of rheumatic heart damage. At the age of 24, he began to develop shortness of breath (dyspnea) on exertion and a distressing cough. He worked in a factory, packing pickles, a relatively easy job, and yet became so dyspneic that he had to sit down on a barrel to continue his work. He lived in a small house heated by a coal stove and brought up coal from the cellar for the stove in a coal scuttle. This exertion caused marked dyspnea. Frequently, he reached the stage where, when he washed his face and hands after work, he had to stop and sit down before he could dry them.

After three or four weeks, he came to the author as a physician, not knowing that I was beginning to use alpha tocopherol. He was one of those treated in the first year of our investigation of the use of alpha tocopherol in treating heart disease. We had not yet discovered that many such patients cannot tolerate large doses so we started him on 300 units a day from the beginning. He was completely well in three days and had changed his job and was "cutting sand" in the local foundry—a very hard job. We were both astonished, and I found it very nearly unbelievable. It was some time later before I realized how very lucky we both were. He was one of those who could tolerate 300 units from the beginning of treatment.

He was still working at the foundry when he was presented, some four months later, to a group of cardiologists and internists, who attested to the accuracy of the diagnosis and their amazement that he could do such work. His only treatment was alpha tocopherol.

He presented another peculiarity of alpha tocopherol therapy in chronic rheumatic heart disease. After two years of treatment he stopped taking his medication. It was a full six months before he began to develop the symptoms of cardiac failure again, even though he continued to work at the foundry. He was started back on 300 units of alpha tocopherol, since, although we had by now discovered the danger of such a large initial dose, he had responded to it originally. Again he was apparently well in four days. This is contrary to our usual experience in coronary heart disease in which the value of the drug is dissipated in as little as three days.

Obviously, it would be highly desirable to be able to predict which patient could tolerate 300 units initially. So far no criteria have been discovered or developed, and so we must play safe and begin with the small initial dose and gradual increase—90 units a day for a month, 120 units for a month, then 150 units.

The *New England Journal of Medicine* (Volume 279, no. 22, November 28, 1968) carried an article on "Edema and Hemolytic Anemia in Premature Infants, A Vitamin E Deficiency Syndrome" by Ritchie, Fish, McMasters, and Grossman in which this same time interval for the development of clinical results is stated and in which the necessity of a properly standardized product is mentioned. To quote:

"Serum tocopherol level. The serum tocopherol rose to the adequate level of 0.4 mg. per 100 ml. or above within one to three weeks after institution of vitamin E therapy and reached a mean of 0.67 mg. per 100 ml. (range of 0.51 to 0.98) in four to six weeks.

"Clearing of edema. The edema of all sites, and the associated symptoms, cleared completely within a month of the initiation of vitamin E therapy."

This article also states that oral iron negates the effect of vitamin E.

In the light of the far-out theory of some cardiologists that polyunsaturated fatty acids are so desirable, the findings in this paper are certainly timely. "In animals and man, the amount of vitamin E requisite to prevent deficiency has been shown to rise when the polyunsaturated fatty acid (PUFA) content of the diet is increased." Uncontrolled, unthinking increase of polyunsaturated fats in the human diet may well increase the incidence of coronary heart disease in patients and have an adverse effect in all other types of heart disease! They will interfere with the treatment of cardiac patients by alpha tocopherol, since much of the tocopherol will be used up in preventing oxidation of the fats.

We, here in Canada, have been very much interested in the participation of one of our biochemists currently on the staff of the Hospital for Sick Children in Toronto, Dr. David Turner. It was his research which revealed why earlier spacemen, up to and including the Borman flight, had suffered a loss of 20 to 30 per cent of their red blood cells during flights and thus became anemic and fatigued. The reason: a lack of vitamin E in the prepared foods carried by the astronauts. On the Apollo 10 flight, astronauts took vitamin E, and the breakdown of the red blood cells was prevented. They suffered no red cell loss. Two interesting comments made by Dr. Turner in a TV interview were these:

He said that the solution was a guess but that it came to him because he had been in London, Ontario (the site of The Shute Institute), when two London doctors had claimed medical value for vitamin E and, secondly, that the present popular fad for replacing animal fats by the polyunsaturated form led to a decrease in utilizable and necessary vitamin E and that such patients should be given increasing vitamin E. He made the usual mistake, so common in scientists who have had no practical experience with the substance, of stating that vitamin E is in rich supply in normal diets. Vitamin E is, but alpha tocopherol, its only medically potent fraction, just is not.

Specific cases continue.

One worth mentioning is that of a 32-year-old woman, seen ten months after delivery of her first and only child. As this is being written, this child is due to graduate next month in Honour Arts at a Western Canadian university.

At the age of 29, before marriage and while teaching school, this woman had one attack of cardiac decompensation with auricular fibrillation. This was diagnosed as due to chronic rheumatic heart disease. On digitalis and bed rest, the rhythm returned to normal, the failure disappeared, and she returned to her teaching. She married a man who soon afterwards went overseas. On his return, they decided because they were now both over 30, that if they were to have a family they should begin at once. However, mindful of her one episode of auricular fibrillation and failure, they wished to be reassured that it was safe for her to become pregnant. They, therefore, consulted a cardiologist and an obstetrician—both certified in their specialties, holding teaching posts at the university, and well regarded in this largest of Canadian cities. Both assured her that it was safe to proceed and that they would "watch her through," whatever that means.

The result was that seven days after delivery she started to fibrillate and went into deep failure. Under the care of her predelivery cardiologist, she tried to carry on in the home with the help of friends and her husband. The husband was trying to start his own business and was frustrated to the point of anger by the necessity of helping at home and store. By coincidence, recently, another much more recent patient recalled this case. She was one of the friends who attempted to help. She described the chaos and confusion of the household with an active infant and his invalid mother. She had furniture and equipment for looking after the baby at table height, since she was unable to lift the baby.

She came to us after ten months of this, in extreme failure and indeed, with our limited experience, we were sure we could not help her. She agreed to stay in the city and to attend the clinic daily. We started her on 300 units of alpha tocopherol a day, but she became rapidly much worse. We then started her over again on 75 units per day, with gradual increase, and her condition began to improve. Within six months, while ambulatory all this time, her failure disappeared, and she was able to look after her baby, her home, and her husband.

Now, after 20 years, still fibrillating, she is an officer in her university alumnae and the Ladies' Aid of her church and sings in the choir. She has had the care of invalid parents, has moved twice as her husband gained promotions in a large company, and, at 53, is considering giving up some of her social obligations. She will cross the continent next month to see her only son graduate from university.

Understanding the mode of action of alpha tocopherol in chronic rheumatic heart disease depends upon a knowledge of the pathology of the disease, as well as the many actions of the drug. The rheumatic fever episode or episodes that precipitated the cardiac damage consisted of multiple submiliary granuloma affecting the valves and the heart muscle both. Small areas of heart muscle die at the site of multiple Aschoff bodies, the most typical rheumatic granuloma. The resultant scars may be very numerous and certainly decrease the functional level of the myocardium. The healing of these lesions in the valve is effected by vascularization and scar-tissue formations. These processes continue throughout the lifetime of the patient, until the changes have reached the point where the heart can no longer function normally under normal conditions of living.

Of course, there are other factors involved. If the patient lives long enough he will inevitably develop a significant degree of coronary artery disease with consequent diminution of blood supply to the myocardium already damaged by rheumatic heart disease. The two insults to the myocardium add up to too much. Then, too, the continuing damage to the valve leads to a difficult mechanical state, which along with the muscle damage, adds up to a breakdown of cardiac function and the beginning of a failing circulation.

Of course, incidental factors may precipitate failure, pregnancy being one well-known example. Overwork, acute infections, or an accident are other such examples.

For many years, the fact that such patients showed obvious abnormalities in heart sounds, due to the damage to the valves, led to over-concern with this factor alone. Then for a time the focus of attention was the myocardium, since it was obviously impossible to alter the valvular damage. Then again, attention was directed chiefly to the valvular abnormalities when the surgeon entered the picture.

However, the patient when he applies for treatment has had a marked degree of damage to the valves for years without symptoms, chiefly because the damaged myocardium has been able to cope with the added load placed upon it by valvular incapacities.

Alpha tocopherol prevents scar-tissue contraction which we have shown in our burn cases, to be discussed later. However, it also relaxes scar tissue already found in such cases as Dupuytren's contracture and in Peyronie's disease. There has been indirect evidence in our own cases of rheumatic heart disease in that many juvenile cases, treated early and continuously, have shown a disappearance of their murmurs. Presumably the degree of valvular damage was such that murmurs were beginning to be created, but alpha tocopherol treatment reversed the scar tissue formation or contraction, or both.

Therefore, one important action of the drug is to halt the damage in the valve and to slowly, and probably to a widely varying degree, in different cases restore some of the elasticity and function to the valve.

By the decrease in the oxygen need of the heart muscle its function is improved and eventually can once more cope with the added work load due to the valvular damage. Further, the restoration of normal capillary permeability and the establishment of normal gas transfers across the cell membranes halts the degenerative process of the disease and prevents the further, and otherwise inevitable and relentless, progress of the disease.

Many cases of cardiac crippling due to this disease come to mind. The majority of our patients obtain worthwhile help, though a few do not. Some are too far advanced for help of any kind, and this type of case has, so far, been refused by the surgeon. Some improve for a time but then develop further trouble and deteriorate. Some discontinue treatment after a few years, only to inevitably return, but may be by then much harder to treat successfully.

In the long run, the chronic rheumatic heart disease patient has given us some of our greatest satisfaction, partly because he is so often relatively young and a parent of a young family and is so badly needed.

One case I remember well is that of a 47-year-old man, a laborer and a physical exercise devotee, who developed a pain in the left shoulder and a rapid irregular heartbeat when he lifted an 800-pound pipe out of a truck on his left shoulder. He became short of breath, developed an ache in the left side of his chest, and suffered "black-outs" on exertion.

He was told he had an irregular heart and had developed heart failure. He was given digitalis and told to take it easier at work.

On examination, his heart was enlarged to the left; his heart rate was 60, with auricular fibrillation; he had a trace of pitting edema, and the murmurs of mitral stenosis.

Treatment consisted of 25 mgs. twice a day of Hydrodiuril, a diuretic which was discontinued after six months; digitalis sufficient to keep his apex rate at approximately 75 per minute, and the routine alpha tocopherol dosage of 90 units a day for a month, 120 units a day for the second month, and 150 units thereafter. After three and one-half months he was definitely better and was working steadily, but still had dyspnea with heavy work.

After five months he was able to do much heavier work, and after nine months he felt perfectly well.

Eleven months after beginning treatment, he was injured at work and developed phlebitis, which yielded promptly and completely to 450 units of alpha tocopherol in four days.

He has been perfectly well ever since. He still has auricular fibrillation, the rate controlled with digitalis. In January, 1966, his dosage of alpha tocopherol was raised to 300 unit. successfully.

CHRONIC RHEUMATIC HEART DISEASE

This case is included for two reasons. This man developed auricular fibrillation and congestive heart failure in 1959, yet during the years 1962 to 1968, he worked as a laborer laying water pipe for the water works department of a city. His foreman was a religious fanatic and after a disagreement on religion made sure this patient did all the heavy work. Such work as he had to do called for a man of unusual strength. Secondly, as mentioned, he is a physical exercise "nut" and does push-ups, knee bends, etc., before work and before going to bed. He's fantastic! He's 57.

Fortunately, since the foreman has retired, he has had a better and much easier job during the last year.

A single woman, aged 48, was first seen on May 2, 1962. She complained of extreme tiredness, shortness of breath on climbing stairs, edema of both ankles by evening, and severe muscle cramps in both feet.

She had two attacks of chorea (involuntary movements) as a child. She developed pneumonia at the age of 20 and following convalescence from this returned to work, but collapsed at her place of employment. She was seen by her doctor who referred her to the dean of cardiologists in Canada. He made the diagnosis of rheumatic heart disease, and she was put to bed for several months. She was able to work only six months from the age of 20 to 28.

She did regain ability to work for the next 20 years by living a carefully restricted life. However, in the weeks before coming to me she had developed fast heartbeat and palpitation and the edema, etc., previously mentioned.

On examination her heart was found to be considerably enlarged with particular enlargement of the left auricle. Her hemoglobin was 50 per cent (anemia), her blood pressure 120/80, pulse regular at a rate of 72. She had a little edema of both ankles and moderate to small varicosities superficially in both legs.

She was started on the routine dosage schedule of alpha tocopherol — 90 units for four weeks, 120 units for the next four weeks, and then 150 units a day. For the first month she took all this in a single dose and an iron product in a single dose 12 hours later to avoid interference with her vitamin E. On this schedule her hemoglobin rose to 82 per cent, and she was symptom-free.

In November, 1962, she developed a broncho-pneumonia with pain in her chest. On December twenty-eighth at 11 p.m. she developed a right-sided femoral artery thrombosis with numbness in the leg. She was immediately hospitalized, and on examination it was found that she had developed auricular fibrillation with râles in the base of both lungs. Her leg was cold and white, and there was no pulsation in the arteries below the inguinal ligament.

Her alpha tocopherol dosage was doubled, she was digitalized by the rapid method, and within hours the leg had returned to normal with a return of pulsation in all palpable vessels. She was discharged four weeks after admission.

She was able to return to work in two more weeks and remained quite well for the next five years. On her regular check-up on May 9, 1967, she reported blood in her stool. She was immediately sent to a surgeon who found a carcinoma (cancer) of the upper third of the rectum. Microscopically, the small invasive tumor did not penetrate the muscle layer, and the surgeon felt sure that there would be no recurrence.

The cardiologist assigned to watch her while in this hospital does not "believe" in vitamin E, and although the surgeon promised me she would be on her vitamin E while in the hospital, except for the day of the operation, she did not receive it. The result was a large area of acute thrombophlebitis in the right leg on the fourth post-operative day. The relatives called me, I went into town to see her, telephoned her surgeon who hastened down to the hospital, and restored her alpha tocopherol. She made an uneventful recovery and was discharged three weeks after surgery.

She has done very well since, and today was in for her regular check-up. After more than seven years of attendance here, she volunteered the information that she felt very well, better than for a long time.

CHAPTER 7. *THE ELECTROCARDIOGRAM*

THE ELECTROCARDIOGRAM IS AN auxiliary instrument in the diagnosis of cardiac disorders, but its limitations must be understood and its rightful place realized. It is often quite normal in the presence of gross cardiac abnormality, and the abnormal patterns can occur in patients with perfectly normal hearts. It therefore gives false negatives as well as false positives.

Moreover, in coronary heart disease, many tracings submitted to several cardiologists will produce widely different interpretations. Those called normal by some will be interpreted as showing evidence of heart damage by others. Of course, all will agree on the significance of certain specific changes in many tracings.

Dr. D. Short (**113**) of the Aberdeen Royal Infirmary investigated 206 consecutive cases of suspected mild or subacute coronary attacks. Of 36 patients who were later proven to have had a myocardial infarction, the initial electrocardiogram showed the infarction in only one quarter. Half of these initial electrocardiograms showed abnormalities which did not indicate infarction, and the balance had no abnormalities.

In this study 100 electrocardiograms, along with the clinical notes originally submitted with the requisition, were submitted to 20 cardiologists. This group agreed entirely on 21 of the 100 electrocardiograms and most (90 to 95 per cent) agreed on another 23. A majority agreed on 77, but there was great disagreement on 23.

Of course, this is a very serious matter, since a firm diagnosis of coronary occlusion was made in 49 cases by one cardiologist, but with the same tracings, on only 23 by another in contrast to 40 made originally!

Think what that variation meant to the patients concerned. The reverse is also worth dwelling upon, since 27 were said to be normal by one cardiologist, but only 14 by another!

Thirty per cent of the 206 cases had a final diagnosis of something in the heart other than infarction. In more than half of these the electrocardiogram was abnormal.

Dr. Short concluded that "The limitation of the electrocardiogram lies in the fact that a single tracing recorded early in an attack of myocardial infarction frequently shows no absolutely diagnostic features, whereas in attacks not due to myocardial infarction, the electrocardiogram is often grossly abnormal on account of previous infarction or other cardiac disease."

The diagnosis of acute rheumatic heart disease is made by the history of a preceding streptococcal infection and the clinical picture of a migrating acute arthritis, an increased sedimentation rate, etc. Most patients show transient electrocardiographic changes, typically a prolonged ST interval and may show peaked P waves, but these changes are usually missed.

The diagnosis of chronic rheumatic heart disease is made on the basis of history and the typical murmurs as heard with the stethoscope. The electrocardiogram is usually normal if no auricular fibrillation has developed.

The diagnosis of hypertensive heart disease is made with the blood-pressure cuff. The electrocardiogram may show left axis deviation.

In coronary atherosclerosis, with angina, even severe angina, the diagnosis is made purely on the patient's history, perhaps reinforced by the effect of nitroglycerin on the attack. The electrocardiogram is commonly normal, although temporary changes may occur during an attack of pain.

In coronary occlusion, as explained above, the initial electrocardiogram may be normal and the patient told that he does not have the condition. He may even be allowed to drive home to a distant city, as in several of the cases seen here. Usually, the electrocardiogram will show some diagnostic sign by the fifth day if it is going to. Then, too, patients with definite occlusions, with infarction, often appear weeks or months later with normal electrocardiograms, but with a definite diagnosis having been made elsewhere. This can be very confusing unless adequate electrocardiographic tracings were taken at appropriate intervals at the time of the occlusion and during hospitalization. This can be of utmost importance, of course, as the following case will illustrate.

This man, aged 43, was seen on June 27, 1949, complaining of angina pectoris. His electrocardiogram was normal. In October, 1947 (20 months previously), while playing badminton in Montreal, he developed pain in his chest and right arm. He sat down for a few minutes and then finished the game. The pain recurred three weeks later. On November 27, 1947, he was hospitalized with the diagnosis of a posterior myocardial infarction from which he made an uneventful recovery. Shortly afterwards, he was offered a promotion, which involved moving to Toronto with his family, the move contingent upon evidence of adequate good health. Consequently, he was sent to another cardiologist, at a different hospital in the same city, who was, incidentally, the head of the medical staff. A tracing taken then was reported in these words, "One can read into this a degree of myocardial change, but I believe the changes are rather insignificant. There is certainly nothing to warrant a diagnosis of any coronary occlusion, and there is nothing very definite to suggest coronary sclerosis or insufficiency."

Please note that he did not bother to contact the previous cardiologist in the same city or ask for the electrocardiogram from the other hospital. He further suggested that his symptoms might be due to gall bladder disease or to duodenal ulcer. X-rays showed a duodenal ulcer, which responded to treatment, and apparently absolved the heart of any complicity in the symptoms.

Of course, everyone was delighted. He received his promotion and moved his family to Toronto.

While skiing in February, 1949, he had a recurrence of chest pain. He was sent to the major hospital in Toronto, and an electrocardiogram taken reported as follows: "ST in CF-IV depressed. T-1 low diphasic and T-4 is low negative. The significance of the depressed ST-4 is unknown. The ST segments in leads I and II are a little low but would pass as within normal limits. Angina or coronary insufficiency can produce such a pattern."

A review of this patient's electrocardiograms obtained from all three hospitals and compared with ours proved that he had, indeed, had a coronary occlusion with a posterior myocardial infarction. While skiing he suffered an occlusion in the opposite artery, with the early changes of an anterior infarction, the two cancelling each other out and leading to a nearly normal electrocardiogram by June, 1949.

Obviously, his care and treatment, after two occlusions involving both anterior and posterior infarctions, differed somewhat from that accorded a man with a little occasional angina.

Nothing yet invented in this atomic and computer age approaches the importance of a careful, detailed history taken by a properly trained physician and that coupled with a careful physical examination and supplemented by whatever laboratory tests he deems wise.

CHAPTER 8. *HIGH BLOOD PRESSURE*

WHAT CAUSES HIGH BLOOD PRESsure? At a recent New York Heart Association conference, the 850 or so experts gathered there had to admit that 95 out of 100 times they did not know. There have been more than 20,000 scientific articles in the last 60 years on the subject of "primary" or "essential" or "idiopathic" hypertension, differing widely as to diagnostic criteria, estimates of its prevalence in the general population, and guesses as to its cause and mortality rate. However, it seems quite clear that most manifestations of the disease are the consequences of, or are made worse by, the presence of raised pressure. Also, the higher the arterial pressure, whether systolic or diastolic or mean, the higher the morbidity and mortality.

There is probably a fair proportion of cases in which glomerulonephritis (a kidney disease) in childhood was a causative factor. Also, some cases in the adult are due to a pheochromocytoma (an operable type of benign blood vessel tumor) and can be surgically corrected. Some cases follow the toxemia of pregnancy.

Hypertension, as a disease, affects about 10 million people in the U.S. Its victims eventually develop organic complications that cut their life expectancy by approximately 20 years. Heredity is vital, since if one parent has it, at least one of a large family will eventually become hypertensive, while if both parents have it, most of their children will also eventually develop it.

In 1964, Dr. Irvine Page wrote accurately that, "Among

the diseases of the heart and circulation, only arteriosclerotic disease of the blood vessels exceeds hypertension as a cause of death." Since that time, during the past five years, the incidence of high blood pressure has been on the increase, yet the mortality rate due to this cause has slowly been falling. In the past 15 years deaths from hypertensive heart disease have decreased by from 50 to 55 per cent. It is no small accomplishment; and thanks for it are due almost exclusively to pharmaceutical research and the development of remarkably effective new anti-hypertensive agents.

In fact, it is these blood-pressure reducing agents that have solved what used to be the trickiest problem in vitamin E treatment of heart disease. The kind of large dosage, 400 to 1,600 units, of alpha tocopherol that has been found most effective in the treatment of coronary thrombosis and myocardial infarction, will usually improve the tone of the heart muscle and so raise the blood in the patient with hypertension. Immediately after a heart attack this may not represent a significant problem since one effect of the attack is to sharply lower the pressure. But where there has been a history of high blood pressure, as occurs in a very large proportion of these cases, in time the pressure will rise once more, and the greater strength of the beat of the improved heart muscle produced by vitamin E will tend to raise the pressure still higher.

Formerly, we were faced constantly with this dilemma. The patient with obvious evidence of coronary heart disease, with a definite hypertension, must have an adequate dosage of the drug. However, in many cases the blood pressure, already too high, would rise still higher. This problem has been neatly resolved by the development of the anti-hypertensive medications. Of the range of these that have become available, I have found chlorothiazide and its derivatives the most useful. Where they are contraindicated, as with existing or latent diabetes, we use the Rauwolfia group, and sometimes if the pressure is high enough and the situation sufficiently critical, we will use the two in combination.

The quick reduction in pressure obtained by use of these drugs and the continuing ability to control pressure with them makes it possible to safely embark at once on a large dosage (from 400 to 1,600 units) of alpha tocopherol and secure a rapid beneficial effect on the heart and the coronary arteries. Ultimately, when sufficient recovery has been made, we will eliminate the hypertensive drugs and find that, in many cases, the blood pressure remains normal or nearly normal without them.

The ability to suspend the use of these drugs instead of continuing them perpetually is no small advantage. It is well known to all doctors that not only these, but all antihypertensive drugs, can sometimes be accompanied by serious complications, particularly under conditions of prolonged use.

One seemingly common result of using the thiazide derivatives is a build-up of uric acid in the system. The excess of uric acid in the blood — hyperuricemia — may be without serious consequences in some patients, while in others acute gouty arthritis, kidney stones, or even kidney collapse may ultimately result. While we are aware of these potential complications, experience has shown that these dangers are minimal in the patient on a large dose of alpha tocopherol.

Although the thiazides do not cause any glucose build-up in the nondiabetic patient, where diabetes exists even as only a tendency or a latency, the thiazides may bring on hyperglycemia, a concentration of glucose in the blood above the normal limit. Inasmuch as the frequent urination brought on by diabetes is easily mistaken for the simple diuretic effect of the drug, it is entirely possible for the diabetes to advance to the stage of severe ketosis before the diabetic condition becomes apparent.

Fortunately, stopping use of the drug will quickly eliminate any enhancement of blood glucose levels that the drug has caused, and the chief danger is that the condition may go too long unnoticed because frequent urination is expected from a diuretic.

Of course, when there is frequent urination and a dehydrating effect for any reason, there is always the possibility of severe depletion of the electrolytes sodium, potassium, and chloride. While this is ordinarily prevented by dietary means, prevention or correction of such deficiencies can become extremely difficult in the presence of a kidney disorder.

There are mental changes that reportedly occur in about 15 to 25 per cent of those treated with Rauwolfia derivatives. They have been few in our own experience, because we do not continue the medication that long. But for those who keep patients more or less permanently on Rauwolfia, there is a high incidence of severe and lasting depression, which strongly resembles involutional melancholia or the depressed phase of manic-depressive psychosis. On occasion, the depressive effect of the drug has led to attempted suicides.

Other mental changes due to Rauwolfia include marked lethargy, frequent nightmares, and sometimes a tremor like that of Parkinsonism.

It is a decided problem that it sometimes takes from three to six months after withdrawal of the Rauwolfia for the mental changes to disappear.

Rauwolfia also poses a very difficult problem at times when the need for surgery may arise. Anesthesia and even minimal losses of blood in such patients result in a profound drop in blood sugar, a danger at any time and marked danger to the patient with coronary heart disease. Angina pectoris, acute myocardial infarction, acute pulmonary edema, and cerebral thrombosis have been reported as the result of such hypotensive episodes following the administration of anesthesia.

The side effects of these very good and highly effective drugs make it highly desirable that their use be discontinued as soon as possible.

Before the advent of these antihypertensive drugs, we made the disconcerting discovery that the larger dosages of alpha tocopherol would elevate the blood pressure in about one-third of the hypertensive patients, often to a marked and, of course, dangerous degree. However, it would neither lower nor raise the pressure in another one-third and thus not reduce the dangers implicit in the hypertensive, while it would lower the blood pressure, occasionally to normal, in the other one-third. Obviously, then, if the full use of the blood-pressure lowering effect of these new drugs is added to alpha tocopherol, it is possible in all cases to initiate adequate treatment at once and so obtain the full benefit of the alpha tocopherol. However, those cases in which the pressure would drop to a lower or normal level were hidden by the use of the antihypertensive drugs, as were also the middle third in whom the blood pressure had not been elevated.

Therefore, when the desired clinical improvement has been obtained, the cautious decrease in the dosage of the antihypertensive drugs will reveal the fact that they are no longer necessary in approximately two-thirds of the hypertensives treated.

Where there is no emergency or the hypertensive drugs are contraindicated, it is possible to revert to a technique that we used to use before the advent of chlorothiazide and its companion drugs. It was based on the observation that small doses of alpha tocopherol will relieve spasms in the arteries and, by reducing the peripheral resistance in doing so, may lower an elevated blood pressure. We thus aimed at obtaining this effect first before increasing the dosage to the larger therapeutic levels that would benefit the heart itself.

In this method, the initial dosage of alpha tocopherol is no more than 90 international units a day and, perhaps, even less for a period of one month. For the second month, the dosage is raised only slightly to 120 international units, succeeded by 150 units in the third month.

Subsequent increases are handled very carefully until adequate therapeutic levels are reached.

With this routine, many patients responded beautifully by a lowering of pressure, which did not become elevated again when therapeutic levels were reached.

The treatment is obviously not as satisfactory as that which utilizes the hypertensive drugs, but there are cases in which the drugs would simply be too dangerous to use. In such a case, it is well worth trying. Results can be and have been very good at times.

CHAPTER 9. *CONGENITAL HEART DISEASE*

CONGENITAL HEART DISEASE — the birth of babies with structural defects of the heart — is by no means rare; and the paucity of medical writing on the subject was more because there was no treatment for the affliction than because it was not recognized as a problem. Approximately 25,000 children — from 0.3 per cent to 0.5 per cent of all live births — are born yearly with abnormal hearts in the U.S. alone. This figure does not include that other substantial number in which abnormal structure of the heart may occur along with other structural abnormalities, as happened in great numbers during the thalidomide tragedy.

With the vast forward leaps that have come in cardiac surgery in recent years, however, it has become possible to effect complete surgical cure in many types of congenital heart disease, in a few of them even without appreciable operative risk. Thus, it is no longer enough to make the nonspecific diagnosis of "congenital heart disease." It is important to make a specific diagnosis of the precise type and of the severity of the heart anomaly.

Among the various kinds of congenital heart disease that can occur, there are at least three which allow of complete surgical cure with little operative risk. They are *patent ductus arteriosus*, a wide open condition of a fetal blood vessel which connects the pulmonary artery directly to the descending aorta, resulting in the recirculation of arterial blood back through the lungs; *coarctation of the aorta* which is a malformation causing stricture and narrowing of the aorta; and *interatrial septal defect*, in which there is an abnormal opening, large or small, between the right and left auricles.

Other congenital defects of the heart can also be treated surgically, although the operative risk is greater than in the three conditions mentioned above. Thus, if there is any reason at all to suspect that there might be a congenital defect of the heart, a thorough cardiological investigation of the newborn has become a matter of prime importance.

While many cases remain unexplained, three specific causes of congenital anomalies are known and make painstaking check of the newborn heart obligatory.

The best known, of course, and perhaps the prime cause, as well, is rubella — German measles. Occurring during the first two months of pregnancy, rubella will lead to congenital defects including those of the heart in most babies. If the mother should contract the disease later in her pregnancy, the danger is diminished, but by no means eliminated. Occurring any time during pregnancy, rubella demands a suspicious and searching examination of the child's heart.

Drugs taken by the mother during pregnancy may also cause abnormalities in the fetus. The best-known example of this, by far, is the large number of abnormal babies born to mothers who were given thalidomide to relieve morning sickness. Even aspirin, however, has experimentally been shown to be capable of causing congenital anomalies, and the spectrum of drugs that might possibly damage the development of the fetus has now become so wide that many physicians will refuse to prescribe any drug during the first trimester of pregnancy except in extreme emergency.

A third cause for many congenital anomalies has been well established by Dr. Evan Shute, who has also shown convincing proof that many such cases can be prevented.

Except where there has been reason to suspect that congenital heart disease might develop and a well-trained cardiologist has made an examination with the stethoscope at birth, in many young patients the defects may be minor and the condition unrecognized during the first few years of life.

It will not be overlooked, of course, in the presence of cyanosis, increasing when the infant cries. This condition is due to admixture of venous and arterial blood through an abnormal pathway between the two systems. The oxygen saturation of the blood leaving the lungs is usually normal, but it becomes mixed with venous blood before it arrives at the site of the right-to-left shunt. When the equivalent of approximately five grams per 100 ml. of unsaturated hemoglobin is present in the arterial blood, the blueness or cyanosis in nail-beds, mucous membranes of the cheeks, and in the lips becomes clinically evident. In some cases, though, cyanosis is not obvious, and in others there is none.

Victims of congenital heart disease show symptoms in varying degrees, depending upon the type and severity of the abnormality. Most cyanotic cases develop polycythemia (an excess of red blood cells), and these patients have, therefore, an increased danger of forming clots leading to cerebrovascular thrombosis. Especially is this true if dehydration, for any reason, occurs.

In children with congenital heart defects there is a greatly increased incidence of infection, particularly respiratory. Bronchitis and pneumonia, as well as frequent colds, are the rule. Many little patients breathe easier and are more comfortable if they rest in a squatting position. Characteristically they will often sit in a chair with knees drawn up and clasped by their hands. Such children may be very uncomfortable if made to stand up straight, or if placed on an X-ray table and tilted backwards.

Ten per cent of all cases of subacute bacterial endocarditis occur in cases of congenital heart disease. This complication, which is an ever-present danger, was invariably fatal until the advent of antibiotics.

Finally, brain abscess, while not common, is another danger that is always present in these patients.

Even those medical men who treat these patients without alpha tocopherol are agreed that how such cases are handled depends upon an accurate assessment of the surgical risk, the possibility of worthwhile improvement from surgery, and the prospects for life and health with medical management alone.

Of course, we agree and insist that all our patients are

adequately investigated, diagnosed, and evaluated and that all cases of *patent ductus arteriosus, coarctation of the aorta* and *atrial septal defect*, all of which can be surgically corrected with low risk, submit to operation.

Years ago, when the question first arose of treating patients with congenital heart disease, we embarked upon their care very gingerly, since it was perfectly obvious that no medication taken by mouth could have any ability to correct a birth defect. Even though it cannot alter a defective structure, however, the oxygen-sparing action of alpha tocopherol and its antithrombin activity are of great value in those cases which cannot be treated surgically. It is also the ideal treatment preoperatively and postoperatively for all those undergoing surgical repair.

We have seen cases of maximal cyanosis, which it should be remembered indicates insufficient oxygen in the blood, as well as many with moderate to mild degrees. In every case, the cyanosis was decreased with an adequate dosage level of vitamin E. In the mild to moderate cases, the cyanosis disappeared. Coincidentally, the "squatters" ceased to squat, there were no episodes of cerebral thrombosis, the number of upper respiratory infections lessened, and, among most of our patients, these symptoms are no more frequent than among the "normal" members of the population. Many of our patients lead normal lives, and they survive.

For any doctor interested in a rapid evaluation of the clinical effectiveness of alpha tocopherol, I suggest that he treat:

1. a case of fresh, acute thrombophlebitis;

2. a case of fresh, acute glomerulonephritis;

3. a case of fresh acute rheumatic fever; or

4. a case of mild to moderate cyanotic congenital heart disease.

He will find the effects unmistakable and very likely beyond his expectations.

Occasionally, patients with congenital heart disease develop rheumatic heart disease as well, following an episode of rheumatic fever. When this is suspected, we immediately become more cautious in treatment and start such patients on smaller initial doses of the drug. Otherwise, these patients seem to tolerate the larger doses very well indeed. A trial dosage level of 300 units a day is about right. In the younger patients, this may be adequate, although we tend to increase the amount of alpha tocopherol at six-week intervals until satisfied that the maximum response for that particular patient has been obtained.

The older patient is usually begun on 600 units a day, with increases if necessary at six-week intervals, until we are satisfied that no further improvement will be obtained.

Up to the time of the publication of "Alpha Tocopherol (Vitamin E) in Cardiovascular Disease" in April, 1954, the Shute Clinic had treated 28 cases. Twelve or 43 per cent became completely asymptomatic, seven or 25 per cent showed a very worthwhile improvement, two were helped, one helped but little, and three died. Two of these fatalities were adults, both *in extremis*. Both were helped initially, but they soon died. One, who had been started on our slow regime which does not help or give protection until after the third month, died on the thirtieth day of treatment. The second, who seemed to be doing very well, died in his sleep on the fortieth day — his dose 300 units a day. The first of these did not have time to respond to treatment; the second nearly made it. The third death could be laid at the door of a university cardiologist who, somehow and for some strange reason, persuaded the parents of a child, who had become perfectly well on alpha tocopherol, to stop using it.

Since then, a third adult has died under rather unusual circumstances. She had become much better on alpha tocopherol, yet was still somewhat cyanotic and dyspneic. Her one ambition in life was to have a child of her own, and in spite of all contrary arguments made by every physician who saw her and by her husband, she insisted on becoming pregnant. She had several miscarriages, one while under our care. Her last pregnancy was somehow maintained to term by an excellent local obstetrician. She delivered easily. The obstetrician brought the child to her after the cord was cut. She looked at her child, smiled a beautiful, happy smile, and was dead. We don't know how her pregnancy was maintained, or whether anything antagonistic to her vitamin E was used or actually the cause of her death. Air embolism was most unlikely. Embolism from the pelvic veins was a stronger possibility. There is also a distinct possibility that the work of delivery in a prone position was just too much for her heart.

The following are representative histories of three of these original cases and one or two seen more recently.

The first is a woman, aged 28, who first was seen on September 29, 1948 (approximately 21 years ago). The doctor who delivered her thought there was some abnormality of her heart, but she seemed to develop normally until the age of 13, at onset of menses. As is well known in the natural history of congenital heart disease, this is the event which often precipitates symptoms. On the advice of her physician she stopped school and stayed at home doing light household chores. Her heart would pound and beat rapidly on any exertion. At the age of 20 she took a business course and worked for five years during which she felt very well, then had to stop because any exertion, such as walking upstairs or uphill, gave her rapid heartbeat, shortness of breath, and palpitation.

Her lesion was an auricular septal defect. There was some enlargement and characteristic deformity of the heart.

Her treatment consisted of 300 units a day of alpha tocopherol. On this she became asymptomatic until June of 1957, when she awakened with pounding, spots before her eyes, orthopnea (inability to breath while reclining), and palpitation. The certified cardiologist in the northern Ontario metropolis where she lived insisted on full investigation by a Toronto cardiologist, who informed her that she must have surgery and that otherwise she would be dead within two years.

She elected to go on with her alpha tocopherol, since the

episode that prompted this investigation was the first she had had in nine years.

In 1965, a refresher course and clinic was held in her home town, and the visiting lecturer was the Toronto cardiologist who had supervised her investigation in 1957. He admitted to her that he found her condition hard to believe. She actually felt better in 1965 than ever. She was working normally and had been taking a daily exercise walk of one-half to one mile.

During 1968 she decreased her dosage of vitamin E and soon noticed dyspnea. She raised it back to 300 units a day and was well again until Christmas, when she had a bad cold which developed into a more severe infection, for which she was given antibiotics. (In some patients both fever and antibiotics seem to decrease the effect of alpha tocopherol.) She went down to Florida to convalesce, but either the climate or the aftereffects of her illness and treatment were not helpful. She became dyspneic and developed pain in both arms. So she increased her dosage level to 375 units a day and rapidly improved. When last seen, April 14, 1969, she was once more perfectly well. She is now 49 years old.

The second case is that of a boy, aged two and one-half years, when seen November 3, 1950, with the diagnosis made, after complete investigation in Detroit, of pulmonary artery stenosis and interventricular septal defect. A heart murmur was discovered at birth, at three months he was hospitalized with a respiratory infection, and he was in an oxygen tent for five days.

He was not too susceptible to such infections, however. He was cyanotic only on exertion, but could not run or play hard without obvious dyspnea.

X-ray showed a 25 per cent enlargement of the heart, and when he cried he was definitely cyanotic. His electrocardiogram, then and since, has shown a marked degree of right axis deviation with widening of the QRS complex and negative T waves in the right side of the precordial leads. Yet with alpha tocopherol treatment he is now in junior college, lives normally, and plays golf without trouble.

The third case is that of a boy aged ten when first seen on December 29, 1952. He seemed quite normal at birth, but a murmur was detected when he was examined during the third week of life. He became quite cyanotic with activity when three or four years old. He began at this time to assume a squatting position a great part of the time, or to sit in a chair with knees drawn up to his chin. He was able to go to school but was tired out by Thursday. He could ride a bicycle, but only a short distance and could climb stairs only slowly.

This boy was given progressively larger and larger doses of alpha tocopherol as he grew up — beginning with 300 units a day. He now takes 800 units a day. With great difficulty, we have been able to persuade college and university admission departments that this boy was worth educating. He was last seen July 8, 1968. He was feeling "real well." He bowls tenpins without trouble, teaches school and night school and summer school. He has his Master's Degree in Education and should easily obtain his Ph.D. next year.

Another case is a woman who was 37 when first seen in April, 1960. She was as cyanotic as any patient I have ever seen, was obviously very dyspneic, and complained of a "fullness" in her chest. She had always been bothered with palpitation and tachycardia. She was able to walk a bit some days. On other days she could not walk at all.

She was a "blue baby" at birth. She had rheumatic fever at the age of nine years. She developed in 1946 a shadow in her lung, diagnosed as tuberculosis at first, later said to be pneumonia. It probably was tuberculosis, since she developed a full blown case of this disease in 1963 and was four and one-half months in the sanitarium.

On examination her heart was grossly abnormal in shape with marked dilatation of the left auricle. With both rheumatic heart disease and congenital heart disease, the significance of her murmurs was hard to evaluate. However, she had a loud systolic at aortic and mitral areas, louder at the aortic, and a mitral diastolic with a sharp second sound. As stated, she was very cyanotic, and her fingers and toenails showed a marked degree of clubbing and incurvation.

She was started on 300 units a day, thought she was better in the second week, but then developed a cold.

On May twenty-first, I doubled her dose since she was not obviously improved, and she became much less cyanotic. She was very well by April 24, 1961 — "an awful lot better than she used to be."

On 1,000 units a day she improved still further and had still less cyanosis. Since then, she has had a rough time — food poisoning, tuberculosis, thrombophlebitis, and frequent colds. The thrombophlebitis occurred on a large dose of alpha tocopherol and cleared up on 1,600 units a day. However, this was too large a dose for her heart to tolerate, and her dyspnea, pounding, dizziness, and nausea recurred. As soon as the phlebitis cleared up her alpha tocopherol was reduced to 1,000 units a day with some improvement.

CHAPTER 10. *PERIPHERAL VASCULAR DISEASE*

AS THE TERM IS COMMONLY USED, disease of the peripheral blood vessels — those of the leg and foot or arm and hand — is considered as being limited to those particular conditions in which the flow of blood to the extremities is reduced because of some abnormality in their own blood vessels. In actuality, however, there are a number of more remote conditions that are equally capable of reducing the blood supply to an extremity. There is, for example, the not uncommon occurrence of a cervical rib which can exert pressure on the artery passing across it as it is stretched and compressed. The peripheral blood supply can also be diminished by general systemic diseases, such as anemia; polycythemia vera, blood disease involving a disproportionate increase in red cell mass; hypothyroidism; myxedema, and cardiac disease.

Whichever the cause, the symptoms and diagnostic signs of peripheral vascular disease stem from either a deficiency of blood flow while the patient is at rest or a relative deficiency when the affected tissues demand additional blood, or both.

Of the clinical manifestations that are induced by a deficient blood supply to the peripheral blood vessels, the commonest is intermittent claudication.

The onset is gradual. The patient first begins to feel a pain on walking that is annoying rather than extreme. Although it is sometimes felt in the foot or thigh, it is the calf of the leg that is the commonest site of discomfort. As time goes on, the patient shows a markedly limited tolerance to exercise, noting usually that he can walk a relatively constant distance without discomfort, but that then suddenly there is sharp constricting pain in one or both legs and, perhaps, severe fatigue. The trouble occurs faster if he walks faster, and it occurs more readily in cold weather. If the exercise is continued, usually the muscles will become spastic and cramped, although occasionally a patient will discover that, if he continues to walk at a slower pace, the pain is reduced.

The patient quickly learns that he can walk three blocks or one block or no more than 50 paces and then will suddenly feel his symptoms and be unable to go further. If he rests at that point, however, the symptoms are promptly relieved.

When intermittent claudication exists, involvement of the heart is so common that a painstaking cardiological examination is obligatory. The sequence of occurrence will vary, with cardiac ischemia or deficient blood supply occurring months or years before the onset of the intermittent claudication in many, while many others first develop the claudication and only later develop angina pectoris. Although arteriosclerosis is frequently present, it is seldom a general condition, but affects specific areas to greater or lesser degree, while other areas and blood vessels remain free of the condition, or relatively so. However, when there is a serious degree of artriosclerotic involvement in one area, it is usually followed in time by signs of serious involvement in one or more other major areas.

Particularly in heavy smokers, intermittent claudication is frequently the initial complaint in what develops into Buerger's disease or thromboangiitis obliterans. It is a condition that frequently begins as a phlebitis of the lower extremities without any obvious predisposing cause. With or without phlebitis, of course, a heavy smoking habit diminishes blood flow by narrowing the arterial lumen. In Buerger's disease characteristically the leg pains are not for long limited to times of exercise, but rapidly begin occurring at rest as well. The patient is awakened by severe cramping that can involve both calves and feet and must either get upright and walk about or at least must hang his feet over the edge of the bed in order to secure relief. The condition is also recognizable by the very slow growth of the toenails and a tendency of the hair on the dorsum of the toes to disappear. The hands have a tendency to tingle or become numb and are clumsy.

When there is phlebitis, as is often the case, it is both extensive and highly resistant to treatment. It may lead to localized ulceration and sometimes to gangrene, particularly in the toe or an entire foot.

There is also, of course, arteriosclerosis obliterans, and an arterial venous fistula can cause similar symptoms by the admixture of saturated and unsaturated hemoglobin in the admixture of arterial and venous blood.

All are peripheral vascular disease and susceptible to the same treatment.

Our original cases were elderly men with atherosclerotic peripheral vessels with decreased resistance to mild trauma and with consequent multiple small areas of superficial gangrene. Pulsations in the vessels of the area were diminished or absent. Alpha tocopherol led to healing of the lesions and a partial return of pulsation to the vessels. This was very gratifying to the patients, but more so to us, since here was visual evidence of the tissue-sparing action of alpha tocopherol. Such cases were photographed and along with our burn and varicose ulcer cases were irrefutable. They could not be helped by "the force of our personalities," as one cardiologist claimed was the case in our cardiac cases.

The specific actions of the vitamin E which were chiefly active in such cases, of course, are chiefly two — the oxygen-sparing action directly on the tissues affected and the opening up of collateral circulation.

During the last 20 years we have seen many such cases and have done, on more than one occasion, something which most textbooks and most scientific medical articles have said cannot be done. We have restored life to dying tissue proximal to large areas of gangrene on the heels of patients with severe degrees of atherosclerotic ischemic peripheral artery disease. This allowed the gradual sloughing off of the dead tissue and the healing, without contraction, of the tissues underneath.

A characteristic of this oxygen-sparing action of alpha tocopherol, that we keep stressing, is the very wide variation in the degree in various patients. Most patients get satisfactory results; some do not. However, in even the most extreme cases, results can be excellent and very, very few of our patients have come to amputation.

Begg and Richards have reported on 198 cases of intermittent claudication followed for five to 12 years or to death. The over-all mortality was 46.5 per cent, while the mortality at five years was 25 per cent. Most of the deaths were due to cardiovascular disease, usually myocardial infarction. The over-all amputation rate was 7.1 per cent. Claudication, they concluded, indicates atherosclerosis, usually generalized, since the ten-year survival rate is compared with that of patients who had angina or had survived a myocardial infarction, for the results are similar.

Larsen and Lassen reported on the effects of a six-month regime of vigorous daily walks. The patients walked as energetically as possible for an hour, resting when the pain became too great. They were able to increase their walking distance, measured on a treadmill, to three times the original values. These patients were not on alpha tocopherol, and the beneficial effects of exercise were due to increasing collateral circulation.

This, of course, recalls the experiments of Enria and Fererro (25) in ligation of the femoral vein and the demonstration of the rapid and extensive opening up of collateral channels with alpha tocopherol. Similar experiments by Dominguez and Dominguez (27) in artificial obstruction of the femoral artery have shown the same effect in the collateral circulation when alpha tocopherol was administered.

The combination of alpha tocopherol and a planned consistent course of exercise should give still better results in these cases. We have not instituted a regime of heavy exercise in these cases, chiefly because it was necessary to first establish the actual benefit of the alpha tocopherol alone and then to follow up our cases for long-term evaluation of their results.

The value of this treatment has now been confirmed by a group of doctors in the University of Alberta Hospital; by W. M. Toone, (111) of the Veterans' Hospital in Victoria, British Columbia, Canada; but more importantly by Professor A. M. Boyd of the University of Manchester, who reported good results with 1,650 patients and stated that the drug increased the survival rate, a matter of great importance.

Color photographs of a very few of our impossible cases have been published in our book *Alpha Tocopherol (Vitamin E) in Cardiovascular Disease* and in the *Canadian Medical Association Journal*, (Vol. 76, No. 9, p. 730, May 1, 1957).

Case Histories

Male, aged 60, when first seen January 22, 1958.

His original complaint was of angina pectoris and dyspnea of four years' duration. Angina developed after walking one to two blocks. Alpha tocopherol relieved his angina fairly well, although he did continue to experience some attacks occasionally.

On August 27, 1967, he developed pain in the three central toes of his right foot, and they were definitely cyanotic, but by the next day they were white, and there was no digital artery or *dorsalis pedis* artery pulsation. On an increased dose of alpha tocopherol (1,600 units daily) there was gradual improvement, and by October 18, 1967, pulsation had returned to the arteries. He has had no further trouble.

A second patient was seen as an emergency in my office on December 29, 1959, at the age of 63. He had had a coronary occlusion on December 18, 11 days previously. Four or five days before I saw him the left foot became very sore and painful and cold. A small area of darkening appeared on the top of the fourth toe and a small spot on the great toe, with edema and discoloration of the whole foot to the ankle on the left side, with a similar lesion on the first and second toes of the right foot.

The rest of the legs were very cold and white.

On examination, it was obvious that he had suffered a mural thrombus on the left ventricle of his heart under the myocardial infarct. This thrombus had broken loose and had finally become lodged over the bifurcation (fork) of the common iliac arteries, shutting off the blood supply to both legs. There was incipient gangrene of the first, second, and third toes of his left foot.

He was placed in the hospital, with feet protected by wrapping in cotton under a cradle, and started at once on 1,600 units of alpha tocopherol a day. The end result was that both legs were saved, with the loss of the second toe, which became totally gangrenous and was allowed to slough off spontaneously, since obviously, as far as it was possible, insult to the living tissue immediately proximal was to be avoided. Later, it became obvious that he now had a mild diabetes mellitus, easily controlled by Orinase.

An almost impossible coincidence occurred in this patient's later experience. He was at a motel in Florida, one winter two or three years later, where he met another guest who had an almost identical history. He had had a myocardial infarct. He had had a "saddle" or "riding" thrombus; he had been put in hospital and treated with 1,600 units of alpha tocopherol. He had ended up losing the second toe, albeit on the other foot. This patient came from south of Cleveland, Ohio.

Another patient at the age of 43, in the summer of 1949, entered the over-40 race at a Sunday School picnic. Two thirds of the way down the course, he was brought to an abrupt halt with severe cramps in the calves of both legs. After a few days, the pain subsided, but thereafter cramping in the calves of one leg would develop on walking one-half to one block. This patient had been taking 600 units of alpha tocopherol a day for years before this episode and by his own judgment increased it to 1,600 units a day. Within a month he was improved and within six weeks symptom-free. He could walk or run and could walk a long and hilly 18-hole golf course without trouble for the next 18 years — at the end of which period there was a mild recurrence on the golf course. A slight increase in dosage soon relieved the condition completely, and as of now he is completely free of symptoms.

This case illustrates the rapid relief obtained by some patients when given an appropriate dose of alpha tocopherol, by which the oxygen need of the tissues is greatly reduced.

This man, aged 57, seen on January 24, 1969, four months earlier had developed intermittent claudication in the left leg on walking one block. Now symptoms were beginning in the right leg. An artificial artery transplant was suggested by a cardiovascular surgeon, but through his brother he decided to try vitamin E first.

On examination, the feet were pale and cold, the left more so than the right. There was no pulsation in the *dorsalis pedis* artery in either foot and none in the posterior tibial on the left side.

On 1,600 units of alpha tocopherol a day, his feet were definitely warmer in six weeks, and by the end of the third month of treatment he was able to walk half a mile before mild cramping set in. At the end of six months' treatment, pulsation had returned in the left posterior tibial artery.

It should be noted in passing that he was still smoking 20 cigarettes a day.

Another man was 61 when seen on October 18, 1960. He had developed intermittent claudication five years previously and in this time had consulted several specialists with various diagnoses, treatment, and suggestions, including surgery.

His feet and legs were painful and uncomfortable most of the time. On examination, his feet were pale and cold, and there was no pulsation in either *dorsalis pedis* artery.

This man's improvement on 1,600 units of vitamin E a day was spasmodic at first. However, after nine years, he can walk normally without pain. His home is on a ravine, with 165 steps in front, and he can come up 120 steps without a stop.

This case illustrates the value of alpha tocopherol therapy after an aortic transplant, which incidentally did not improve this patient's condition. We have had, similarly, success with chronic rheumatic heart disease patients whose surgery was unsatisfactory or partially satisfactory or in whom there was a regression after several months.

This patient, aged 47, when first seen on December 11, 1968, had had a coronary occlusion, with an anterioseptal infarct, in August of 1966. He had had intermittent claudication for six or seven years and had a Teflon graft inserted on September 11, 1967 with no change whatsoever in his symptoms.

On 2,400 units of alpha tocopherol a day, he can now walk fairly well, about twice as far as he could previously. We anticipate further improvement.

Another patient was aged 62 when first seen on April 25, 1968. He had developed intermittent claudication in 1964, usually on walking one block. In July of 1967 he developed angina for the first time and since then has had it many times on mild exertion or excitement.

On 1,600 units of alpha tocopherol daily he no longer has any angina, can walk any distance if he takes his time, and is well satisfied.

Still another patient is the owner of a large real estate business and is particularly active in selling farms, which means he must walk over many acres of meadow, bush, and cultivated land. He was 53 years old when first seen September 12, 1968. He first noticed difficulty in walking in 1965, and this had increased steadily. Finally, he was able to walk but one block on pavement and a little more on farm properties, and his legs ached continuously after a day's work. He had had angina for ten years and was a known hypertensive.

On examination, there was no pulsation in the right foot and a very weak one in the posterior tibial artery on that side. The left leg showed excellent pulsation in the *dorsalis pedis* artery and weak pulsation in the posterior tibial. By February 10, 1969, he could walk three times as far and by April 9 was able to walk over three farms in the course of his day's work. By June 25, 1969 there was a definite return of pulsation in the right *dorsalis pedis* and improved circulation throughout.

CHAPTER 11. *VARICOSE VEINS*

THE ACCEPTED EXPLANATION OF the occurrence of varicose veins is that in the affected patient, there are constitutionally defective valves. Postural strain, usually of an occupational type, such as in store clerks, nurses, etc., who are perforce on their feet for several hours at a time, is the precipitating factor.

Also, any condition that obstructs venous flow and distends collateral veins over long periods of time, especially pregnancy and pelvic or abdominal neoplasm, will produce varicosities.

Our training was traditional, and so, of course, this explanation was accepted. Therefore, we at first paid little or no attention to the effects of alpha tocopherol on varicose veins. However, when we compared notes and found that our patients were insisting that their varicose veins were getting smaller, we became interested.

My own experience began with a male patient, who on his first visit for a cardiac problem showed me a large varicose vein about 8 inches long inside his left knee. Later, on a subsequent visit, he mentioned that this vein had "disappeared." He must have noticed my smile and look of incredulity. He said, "You don't believe me, do you?" He then exposed the knee, and there was no visible varicose vein. I could palpate the vein but it seemed normal in size.

A second convincing case was that of a girl in her middle twenties, a member of a large family, many of whom had been patients of mine for years. She asked me to give her vitamin E for her veins, since she was about to be married and didn't want to walk down the aisle with her legs as they were. Obviously, this was in the days of short skirts and sheer stockings! I refused, since the synthetic product we were using at this time was very expensive — 57 cents per 100 units — and obviously also, no drug should be used indiscriminately. Certainly mere vanity was not an adequate reason for treating a patient. I explained this point of view and said that it would be a different matter if she had had any heart trouble. Then she said, "Well, I am supposed to have a damaged valve." She had at that time asymptomatic chronic rheumatic mitral stenosis, so I did treat her for her heart. She was delighted with the effects on her veins and walked happily down the aisle at her wedding. She has remained a patient, has no family, has beautiful legs, and her heart, except for one brief episode, has given her no trouble.

Since these experiences, we have treated patients with varicose veins, with and without previous surgery, with gratifying results. However, the reasons for treatment have been not to shrink the varicosities, but to reduce the symptoms. The distended and torturous veins cause a chronic venous stasis which produces edema, stabbing and aching pain, and, if severe enough and prolonged enough, indolent ulceration, overgrowth of connective tissue, and occasionally, hemorrhages or ecchymosis, leakage of blood under the skin. The ulceration is a condition we have long treated successfully with alpha tocopherol, and, of course, this was our initial interest. It was a bonus to us, however, that the treatment of varicose veins almost always completely relieves the pains and aches by decreasing the oxygen need of the tissues involved; by opening up effective collateral circulation, it also relieves the edema.

Any patient who is content with comfort and doesn't care too much about the appearance of her legs, especially now that stockings are available which give gentle elastic pressure and support and look good, will be satisfied with her response.

Most such patients resist surgical intervention to remove

the affected veins; and we explain to our patients the results with surgery.

The Canadian Medical Protective Association annually warns doctors to consider the operation of the ligation and stripping of veins as "one of the most potentially dangerous any patient may have to undergo because of the irreversible results which generally follow error . . . It is only part of the answer to say that vein stripping should be done only by skilled, experienced surgeons . . . it can be demonstrated that skill alone is not enough, as witness the fact that some of these difficulties have arisen at the hands of the most highly skilled and widely respected practitioners."

Recurrence rates are high after surgical treatment. The etiology of varices is obscure. Accurate and adequate ligation of all communicating veins may still not prevent recurrence because of pre-existing and continuing deep vein incompetence not amenable to surgical correction. There can be no guaranteed permanent cure of this condition. Complications of varicose vein surgery may run as high as 52 per cent, the results bad in four per cent and only fair in 18 per. cent. (Editorial and article by Phillips in the *Scottish Medical Journal* 9: 357, 1964.)

Brown *et al* in the same journal earlier (6: 322, 1961) reported that of 107 limbs with high ligation 59 per cent showed recurrence of the varicosities, and 89 per cent of these were due to incompetent communicating veins. In only 44 of the 107 legs were the results clinically satisfactory.

Contrast this with alpha tocopherol therapy:

One woman patient was aged 35 when first seen on January 26, 1961. Following her first pregnancy, she had developed varicose veins, which had become worse after the second pregnancy. In 1954 she had had vein ligation with some initial benefit, but by October, 1960, her varicose veins were worse than originally. She had them "stripped" by an excellent vascular surgeon with multiple incisions along the courses of the veins in both legs. The result was a singularly unsightly leg with deep hollows at the site of the incisions where all the subcutaneous tissue seemed atrophied.

She had had rheumatic fever at the age of 12 and had been confined to bed for several weeks at that time.

Her legs were cold but not particularly painful. However, she was told that her veins would have to be "kept down" by subsequent operations.

A complication in her case was a duodenal ulcer, which had hemorrhaged severely in 1955 and October, 1959, and recurred again in March of 1969, requiring three transfusions, so her treatment with alpha tocopherol was interrupted while she was in the hospital.

Because of the ulcer history and the rheumatic fever history and the typical murmurs of rheumatic heart disease, she was started very gradually on alpha tocopherol—90 units a day for a month, 120 units for the second month, and then 150 units. By August of 1961 she stated that her legs felt much better. However, her veins were beginning to show some recurrence of the varices, so her alpha tocopherol was gradually raised to 300 units a day. On this quantity her legs have steadily improved. There are no more varices, and they now no longer bother her. She has had no recurrence of ulcer symptoms. The hollows in the subcutaneous tissue at the site of incision are definitely filled in to a degree, though still very obvious.

A man, aged 48 when first seen on March 27, 1961, worked all day on the floor of the stock exchange. Gradually varicose veins appeared in both legs, and they ached and cramped at work. He had developed a patch of varicose eczema, secondarily infected with a fungus, which healed when the fungus was cleared up on 150 units of alpha tocopherol prescribed by a nurse who was also a patient of mine. He was advised to have his veins stripped, but reported to me instead, since his wife was also my patient.

On alpha tocopherol, in six weeks his legs felt warmer and had become "no bother at all." He had no pain or ache or cramps. However, the area over the vein previously treated was bothering him again. Alpha tocopherol in vanishing cream was applied to this lesion with "stupendous results." It is now more than eight years since treatment began.

A woman, aged 39 when first seen June 23, 1964, had a mild attack in both legs of thrombophlebitis which accompanied a pregnancy in 1959. This recurred in her left leg again with her last pregnancy in March of 1963. Since that time the left leg would become edematous by night.

On 600 units of alpha tocopherol the edema disappeared in four weeks, and her legs ceased to bother her.

In November, 1964, with another pregnancy, her legs once more began to ache, so her alpha tocopherol was raised to 800 units daily. At this level her legs once more ceased to bother her. She had no more trouble. Her daughter was born on June 27, 1965, and she has had no trouble with her legs since.

A woman, aged 65 when first seen July 15, 1958, had had varicose veins in both legs since her first pregnancy. During the previous four years there was marked discoloration of both ankles and the lower halves of both legs. It had become worse since varicose eczema and an episode of infection from scratching had set in.

This case is remarkable in that she has 16 children, eight boys and eight girls, and raised all 16 on a Western prairie farm. Her legs bothered her all the time, showing extensive varices in both legs, with severe cramping in bed.

On alpha tocopherol these varicose veins of nearly 50 years duration, aggravated by numerous pregnancies, not only ceased to cause symptoms of venous stasis, but diminished greatly in size. She now wears normal nylon stockings and has a nice pair of legs, just like her eight daughters.

A woman, aged 35 when first seen September 4, 1962, first developed varicose veins with her first pregnancy 15 years previously. Her left leg was the more painful of the two, especially since the birth of her second child four years previously. With this second child, she had a thrombophlebitis while in the hospital. Both legs ached continuously, especially as the day progressed.

On alpha tocopherol therapy her legs ceased to bother her by December (after three months' treatment).

A woman, aged 49 when first seen on September 2, 1964, had had several recurring attacks of thrombophlebitis in her right leg for the prior six years. The last attack was in May, 1964; and the leg was still painful if she was on her feet for any length of time.

She had three episodes of pulmonary embolism following a cholecystectomy in June of 1964 at the time of a phlebitis in her right leg. She was a teacher who taught home economics at a technical school.

On 800 units daily of alpha tocopherol her legs were better in six weeks. However, her doctor had put her on iron, and since neither he nor the patient knew that this interfered with alpha tocopherol therapy, the left leg started to pain again. When it was explained that she could only take iron by taking all her alpha tocopherol at once and all her iron eight to 12 hours later, the legs once more became asymptomatic.

Another patient, aged 51 years on August 30, 1960, had had varicose veins since 1930—some 30 years. She had phlebitis in both legs in 1935 and an acute thrombus in 1960. The varices had increased for the past two years and had a dead heavy feeling in them. There was edema of feet and ankles for 20 years.

In 1956 she had an attack of what may well have been a pulmonary embolus and was in bed a few days.

On 300 units of alpha tocopherol a day, the aching was all gone in six weeks. She decreased her dose of alpha tocopherol and bought an inferior brand because it was cheaper. Her legs started to ache again. On a good brand and 600 units a day, her legs ceased to bother her at all.

A woman, aged 52, was seen first on May 1, 1967. She had been bothered with varicose veins since a pregnancy 24 years before, the left leg being the worse. There was a marked degree of varicose eczema in both legs, and there was a fair degree of edema by the end of the day.

On 800 units of alpha tocopherol the eczema and edema cleared up completely, so she stopped taking the alpha tocopherol. The condition recurred, and she started back on treatment. Once more her legs lost the eczema, so she stopped her capsules again, and the eczema took some time to come back. The edema disappeared. She continues to treat her condition off and on, as above, in spite of my attempts to explain the virtues of continuous treatment! I used succinate (succinic acid salt) in this case because of the varicose eczema and the suspicion that there might be an allergic element in the lesion. There is a lessened chance of allergy with the succinate, although I feel that the usual natural form of alpha tocopherol is more potent and useful.

One patient had a combination of varicose veins and a hemorrhagic tendency, the latter also clearing up on alpha tocopherol therapy. She was 46 years old when first seen on November 14, 1961. She would develop large superficial bruises on her arms, legs, and hands particularly, but anywhere on her body in response to the mildest trauma. She had edema of both legs to the knees, due to varicose veins in both legs. These had been injected 12 years previously and ligated two years later. She suffered cramps in her feet and in the calves of both legs at night.

On 600 units of alpha tocopherol and calcium with vitamin D, she was much improved in six weeks; she had no more bruises, no more cramps, no more edema, and no more aching legs. She has been perfectly free of all these symptoms now for seven and one-half years.

Finally, here is the history of a patient included because of the extent of varicosities recurring after ligation and stripping of veins eleven years before and the degree of improvement achieved in a short time on alpha tocopherol therapy.

The operation, bilaterally, involved six incisions in each leg. When I first saw her August 10, 1967, the whole internal saphenous veins system on the right side was involved in multiple large varicosities to the region of the saphenous opening, and she had large varices on the right side of her vulva. The left side showed the same picture, but to a lesser degree. She had a phlebitis in the left thigh during the whole month of January, and in August her right thigh was very painful.

On 300 units of alpha tocopherol a day she was much improved, her legs didn't ache any more, and the phlebitis was clinically cleared in the right thigh.

This patient was a professional seamstress and made all the clothes for herself and her children. Only at the sewing machine did she notice aching and pain in the right thigh and leg. For this reason her dosage was raised to 600 units a day, and she lost all symptoms. Her legs lost the edema, were slimmer and the veins less prominent and not as dark blue in color.

CHAPTER 12. *THROMBOPHLEBITIS*

THERE IS VERY OFTEN A DISTINCtion made between a primary, simple clot, or thrombosis, in the lumen of the vein, without apparent inflammation, which is called phlebothrombosis, and a similar condition, with active inflammation of the wall of the affected vein, which is, therefore, called thrombophlebitis.

Predisposing factors are: (1) reduced flow of blood through the veins (venous stasis) associated, for example, with prolonged bed rest or external pressure; (2) local injury of the endothelium by stretching, contusion, chemicals, or bacteria; and (3) changes in the circulating blood that favor coagulation.

There are also many clinical conditions which may lead to thrombophlebitis, such as myocardial failure, obesity, debility, senility, varicose veins, trauma, and surgery.

The condition can chiefly or entirely affect the superficial veins, those at or near the skin surface, or may affect the deep veins chiefly or entirely, depending to some degree on the condition of the communicating veins. It is a condition that is usually not difficult to diagnose in the superficial veins, but may be very difficult indeed in the deep veins. This accounts for the wide variation in the reported incidence of deep vein thrombosis, since it may be easily overlooked unless carefully sought for in every bedridden or convalescent patient. In view of how often the possibility is not investigated, it may well be supposed that thrombophlebitis is more common than is generally known.

The condition in a patient can be very widespread. It

usually begins in the leg or thigh but may easily occur in or spread to the pelvic veins, particularly in surgical cases. Of course, the main danger is embolism; as the clot disintegrates, many small emboli or a single large embolus can occur. Deposited in the lungs, such emboli can be rapidly fatal or lead to a serious, long-protracted illness.

In recent years there has been a great rise in the incidence of deep vein thrombophlebitis and so of pulmonary embolism. A study in two Oxford, England, hospitals showed that the incidence in 1961 was about five times that of 1952. The mortality rate was also greatly increased, since about one-half of the cases recorded were fatal. The authors advance the possibility that this phenomenon represents merely one facet of an epidemic of thrombotic disease affecting Western society. During the period under review, the number of patients admitted to the hospitals with coronary and cerebral thrombosis had also risen steeply (S. S. B. Gilder quoting the work of Morrell and her colleagues in the *Canadian Medical Association Journal*, Vol. 89, December 21, 1963, p. 1,300).

G. Stringer in the *New York Journal of Medicine* (62: 3423, 1962) reported that among 150 patients, with phlebitis, followed from five to more than 20 years after the initial illness, 25 had recurrences. There were 20 instances of pulmonary embolism among them. The most commonly occurring sequelae were edema, varicosities, and ulceration. Yet the condition is easy to control with vitamin E.

Very soon after our rediscovery of the value of alpha tocopherol in cardiac disease, Dr. Evan Shute treated a case of antepartum (before childbirth) thrombophlebitis with a "lump" the size of a man's fist in the woman's lower thigh, the veins involved extending from mid-thigh to mid-calf with marked edema in the tissues surrounding the affected veins. On alpha tocopherol the mass and cellulitis disappeared in four days, and the patient left the hospital in ten days. On a maintenance dose, there was no recurrence at delivery. Since then, we have treated a great many such patients, and in the fresh acute stage the response is always within 48 to 96 hours and, by that time, nearly complete. Of course, when a patient is seen some days after the beginning of the phlebitic change, the improvement is slower and less likely to be as complete, since, of course, the clot has become organized.

However, by far the most startling and most important effect is that these patients *do not throw off emboli*. We were alert to this danger in our phlebitic cases, but only once have I had a patient throw a pulmonary embolus. This was in the early days of vitamin E therapy, and at this time we were following the old practice of six weeks in bed for a case of coronary thrombosis.

On routine check-up one morning, one such patient was found to have a thrombophlebitis in his left leg. I promptly increased the dosage of his alpha tocopherol. The very next day he suffered a pulmonary embolus. Since I had already increased the alpha tocopherol, I didn't change it, and in two days his pulmonary embolus was gone. He really wasn't very sick with it.

Consider the implications of this treatment. Instead of vigorous and highly dangerous anticoagulant treatment or, if the condition is advancing, the radical surgery still advocated, one just gives the patient vitamin E and keeps him ambulatory.

Dr. Alton Ochsner, famous in his own right as head of the Ochsner Clinic, "the little Mayo's of the South," has long been interested in thrombophlebitis and its prevention and treatment. He was sent a preliminary paper of ours for perusal and apparently decided to try alpha tocopherol. The results were so excellent that he reported them at the International Congress of Surgeons and in the various medical journals, the *Journal of the American Medical Association*, the *Annals of Surgery*, etc., and lectured on the subject at various medical societies. In the *New England Journal of Medicine* (271, 4, July 23, 1964) appears a letter over Dr. Ochsner's signature commenting on an editorial in the June 4th issue of the journal entitled "Thromboembolism — Spring, 1964." He suggests that it is far more important to stress the desirability of prevention of venous thrombosis rather than treatment of the complication, pulmonary embolism. Later on in this letter he states that "in all patients in whom venous thrombosis might develop, for a number of years we have routinely prescribed alpha tocopherol, 100 international units, three times a day, until the patient is completely ambulatory . . . Alpha tocopherol is a potent inhibitor of thrombin that does not produce a hemorrhagic tendency and therefore, is a safe prophylactic against venous thrombosis. . . . The prophylactic treatment is generally simple and safe."

Dr. Ochsner (67) has since stated that since using this form of prophylaxis, *he has not had one single case of pulmonary embolism.* If this is so, he is almost certainly the only surgeon in America in practice more than a year, who can say so.

Currently, there is much in the medical literature about the increased dangers of thrombophlebitis in women taking contraceptive pills, and the case has been fairly well made out, at least in England. However, "the pill" is probably safer statistically than pregnancy or driving an automobile; and certainly nothing will stop the millions of women who rely on and are delighted with it.

These women and their physicians ought to know that, just as every patient whose doctor has put him on a polyunsaturated fat diet needs increased vitamin E, so does the woman who takes the pill. With the simple addition of a vitamin to her diet, she reduces virtually to zero the danger of thrombophlebitic complications. So, also the woman who is convinced by TV advertising that she must use a certain brand of oleomargarine, because it contains polyunsaturated fats derived from corn oil, needs extra vitamin E.

How much is a daily preventive quota of vitamin E? I am not aware that it has ever been computed with any degree of accuracy or with anything like a full knowledge of the nature of vitamin E deficiency disease. When I make what you might call an educated guess it is 200 international units daily for the adult in normal good health.

As a treatment for thrombophlebitis I use an initial dosage of 600 international units daily. Attempts at lower dosages have uniformly had inadequate effects, and in occasional cases I have even seen embolisms occur while the lower dosage was being administered. Six hundred international units of alpha tocopherol a day will result in consistently satisfactory effects.

Unless the diagnostic signs indicate a large number of clots or one that is indeed massive in extent, there is no need to immobilize the patient. With a sufficient dosage of alpha tocopherol — and the sufficiency of the dosage is readily checked and progress confirmed by a rise in the platelet count — the danger of embolism is for all practical purposes eliminated. Although it always exists in theory, I have never seen an embolism occur, once alpha tocopherol treatment has taken hold.

With this treatment clinical improvement should be apparent and confirmed by a rise in the platelet count within two days. If it does not occur as expected, the answer is to double the dosage. I am convinced there is no such thing as a thrombophlebitis that will not resolve with a concomitant rapid increase in the platelet count in response to a high dosage of alpha tocopherol.

On the other hand, if the initial platelet count is normal or nearly so, the response to the same treatment will be slower, and in such a patient I sometimes will start therapy with a dose as high as 800 international units daily.

I believe this phenomenon occurs because, while a fresh fibrin net will trap platelets thoroughly and cause a low platelet count, the older clot will be harder and partially shrunken and will permit more circulating platelets to pass it. Thus a higher platelet count is an indication of a clot that will be more difficult to dissolve.

Treatment of an older clot takes longer, usually, but it will quickly render the lesion quiescent. However, in such cases, once the edema and inflammation have subsided, a residual mass of vein enclosing an organized thrombus can be felt.

Some cases may be quite difficult to handle when a concomitant cardiac condition is present. I once saw a patient, a middle-aged, very obese nurse, with a very extensive acute thrombophlebitis of some days' duration, involving varicose veins of the thigh up to her inguinal region and, therefore, quite possibly extending into her pelvic veins. Examination revealed chronic rheumatic heart disease with mild congestive failure and moderate hypertension. For the phlebitis she required a large dose of alpha tocopherol. For her heart and blood pressure, she couldn't take a large dose.

Fortunately, she was a local patient and could be watched closely and was always at the other end of the phone. Being a nurse, she could describe any condition that might arise. She was given 800 units a day and told that she could almost certainly take that much for five days, but probably no longer. By the fourth day her phlebitis was much improved, but had not disappeared. On the fifth day she developed severe palpitation, fast heartbeat, shortness of breath, inability to breathe, except sitting up, and a cough. Her alpha tocopherol was stopped for two days with, fortunately, little change in the phlebitis. On the third day, 800 units a day was started again since the cardiac symptoms had cleared up. Four days later, the phlebitis was clinically cleared. However, because of the possibility of extension into the pelvic veins and because there might still be some residual, the dosage was unchanged. The next day she called to say that all her cardiac symptoms had returned.

When I went to see her I was surprised to have her open the door for me. I looked at her large legs with prominent varicose veins and asked how it happened that she was apparently well again. She explained that she was the patient's identical twin!

Recovery was complete after the third four-day treatment and before her cardiac symptoms recurred. Thereupon, we instituted proper treatment of her chronic rheumatic heart disease, and there has been no recurrence of the phlebitis.

A letter in a small but excellent medical journal some years ago described two cases of peripheral edema of unexplained origin, not yielding to treatment. Many chemical and blood tests had been run without anything seriously abnormal. Both were in women, one in a teen-ager, one middle-aged. Finally, by luck, the problem was solved. Both had begun to wear panty girdles sometime before their symptoms began, and their removal cured both cases.

I have a patient, a nurse, who has had some trouble over the years with phlebitis in the right leg. One morning she developed phlebitis in the left leg. Since she was taking enough alpha tocopherol to protect the right leg, I was puzzled as to how this could happen, until the modern short skirt helped me solve her problem. Her mother had given her a lovely expensive panty girdle for her birthday!

Because this book is intended to show how an experienced user of alpha tocopherol meets a variety of problems, this case is presented here.

A 63-year-old hairdresser had rheumatic fever at the age of 16, was quite ill at the time, and was kept in bed for one year. On June 13, 1969 she developed thrombophlebitis in her right leg. She was hospitalized for five days and given Butazolidin. There was some decrease in the thrombophlebitis; but all the symptoms were still present, and she was unable to stand on the leg for any length of time.

On June 13th her doctor discovered that her blood pressure was elevated and placed her on Serpasil-hydrochlorothiazide pills.

When seen here on July 7, 1969, her blood pressure was 145/90 and her right leg showed a purplish red discoloration along the course of the great saphenous vein, which could be seen and palpated for ten inches below the knee and which was very tender and obviously thrombosed.

She presented an obvious problem in that she had a damaged rheumatic heart and had recently had hypertension. She was put on 225 mgs. of alpha tocopherol a day (see the precautions outlined in the chapter on chronic rheumatic heart disease and in Chapter XIX, "Tailoring the Dose"). It was hoped that this might be enough to control the thrombophlebitis and not so much that it might precipitate heart symptoms. Then, too, we originally used such a dosage on many cases.

Fortunately, she responded well, although slowly. In two and one-half to three weeks there was marked improvement, and in four weeks all signs of inflammation were gone. There was still a three-inch length of vein that was firm to palpation; but there was no tenderness, no discomfort, and she was able to work. She felt well in herself. Her blood pressure was 140/90 and her pulse 76.

A male patient, aged 45 when first seen April 23, 1969, had had an area of thrombophlebitis inside the knee six weeks previously. He was treated with an anticoagulant and then developed a large subcutaneous hemorrhage a week and a half later. Since he was forced to put more weight on the right leg, the veins on that side were beginning to ache.

This man's varicose veins in his left leg had been tied 11 years before, because they had been large and bulging and the leg ached. The leg was somewhat improved for four or five years, and then gradually the original condition returned and then worsened still further.

When this acute thrombosis occurred he was given the anticoagulant which brought about a definite decrease in the thrombophlebitis. At this point, a specialist was called in to advise upon further prophylactic care to prevent recurrences. He suggested the injection of some substance intramuscularly every six hours for a week or so. The patient then developed a severe sciatica, which has persisted now for five months, causing severe difficulty in walking. Then the hemorrhage in the thigh occurred, so he was transfused with whole blood. Because he had fainted with the pain, he was put in oxygen. Of course, the anticoagulant was discontinued. He was in hospital for another two weeks.

He was seen here six weeks after he was first admitted to hospital. At this time, the left leg was black and blue and swollen and hot behind the thigh and knee over a very large area around the varices and the vein itself. The thrombosis and ecchymosis around the vessel were palpable and visible. His temperature was 99 degrees, his pulse 84.

He was given 1,200 units of alpha tocopherol a day. Two weeks later there was less aching, there was no edema, the subcutaneous hemorrhage was much less apparent, he had no fever, and his pulse rate was 68.

A month later the clot could still be palpated between the two ligations in that area. By August 13, 1969 his leg felt better than it had for years, the hemorrhage was gone and the vein and varices barely visible. He still had difficulty walking, with the sciatica still present, very little improved, and not yielding to treatment.

CHAPTER 13. *ARTERIAL THROMBI*

AS HAS BEEN STATED IN THE INtroduction, the leading cause of death in the civilized world today is thrombi forming in the coronary artery. It must be obvious that thrombi can form anywhere in the cardiovascular tree and that the danger of embolism from such thrombi is, of course, always present. That thrombi in the veins of the extremities and pelvis are now very commonly found in puerperal and postoperative patients and in the chronically ill and bedridden and that the incidence of such thrombi has increased in almost parallel fashion to coronary thrombi is becoming evident (112). Similarly thrombosis of the cerebral arteries is becoming more common.

In all cases of thrombosis, the treatment of choice is alpha tocopherol. In venous thrombosis, treated immediately the diagnosis is made, the results are spectacular; if treatment is begun later, however, it is less so. The vitamin's ability to dissolve fresh venous thrombi is well documented.

In acute coronary thrombosis the direct action of the alpha tocopherol on the clot in the artery is greatly curtailed by the mechanical difficulty of getting the tocopherol to the clot because of the relative and absolute paucity of collateral vessels. Therefore, the clinical evidence of the effect of the drug depends upon the clinical effect on the patient and upon the serial changes in the electrocardiogram. In general terms, it can be stated that the electrocardiogram shows the same serial changes as occur in a typical case not treated with alpha tocopherol, but to a much lesser degree. However, the electrocardiogram recovery is much more rapid and much more complete than in the untreated patient. Clinically, the patient is usually much less ill, and has a quieter convalescence and an unusually rapid and complete recovery.

We think the same to be probably true of the victim of cerebral thrombosis, but neither this nor the direct effect on the thrombus in the coronary artery is susceptible to proof and must, at least at present, remain a clinical impression.

However, there is an interesting analogy between these two situations and the demonstrable effect of alpha tocopherol on burns. If alpha tocopherol ointment is applied to a burn immediately, only that tissue destroyed by the injurious agent is lost. Without alpha tocopherol ointment, the toxic products of the dead tissue destroy the injured but viable tissue beneath, and the burn deepens. Similarly, in the coronary and cerebral accident the zone of injury and the zone of anoxia are invaded by the alpha tocopherol, and the infarct or area of softening is reduced. Recovery, therefore, is more rapid and complete. This is logical, and this we believe to be self-evident.

Embolism is an ever-present danger and one that we have feared in treating coronary occlusions (from mural thrombi under the infarcted area) in our cases of thrombophlebitis and in our cases of chronic rheumatic heart disease with auricular fibrillation. We have had very, very few, indeed, to our great joy.

I can remember but one embolism occurring in a coronary occlusion, and the pulmonary embolus resulting rapidly resolved with very little discomfort to the patient. There have been none in memory in cases of thrombophlebitis and several, but still relatively rare, emboli in chronic rheumatic heart disease with auricular fibrillation.

Two cases of peripheral arterial embolism have been reported elsewhere. One, a riding or saddle thrombus occluding the common iliac arteries in both legs in a case of coronary occlusion, the other an embolus to the right common iliac artery in a patient with chronic rheumatic heart disease with auricular fibrillation.

These cases certainly support our impression that the effect of the alpha tocopherol is directly upon the fresh thrombus itself, as has been demonstrated by several authors in the case of acute thrombophlebitis.

CHAPTER 14. *INDOLENT ULCER*

IN MANY CASES OF VARICOSE VEINS, ulceration eventually occurs. It is usually on the front of the leg, a few inches above the ankle. Often it is initiated by a bump, a blow, or some other mild trauma. However, the extravasation of blood around the veins in this area has usually resulted, over the years in gross staining with iron pigment (hemosiderin) and other pigments from the breakdown of the red cells in the tissue, a virtual tattooing. The pigments induce irritation in the subcutaneous tissues, which leads to changes in the connective tissue, with contraction in many cases, and this collagenosis seems to predispose the area to ulceration even when there is no specific trauma.

Such ulcers are remarkably persistent. Indeed, they tend to spread as the toxic products of tissue breakdown and the usual surface infection destroy fresh marginal cells. Healing forces simultaneously come into play, but the new tissue may in turn break down, giving a typical chronic edge to the ulcer. Very often there is a dilated "sentinel vein" just above the ulcer. The base of the ulcer is usually covered with a soft layer of material made up of fibrin, leucocytes, and *purulent* exudate, often foul-smelling.

Many forms of treatment have been used, often with success. Among them are various antibiotic ointments and support of the edematous surrounding tissue by elastic bandage or Unna's paste bandage to form a soft cast. Many cases have had the sentinel vein tied off or injected, although this maneuver is rarely of much value. When it works, of course, such treatment heals the ulcer once, and it may stay healed. More commonly, though, it breaks down eventually, or new ulcers form in the same area or adjacent to it.

Many such ulcers do not even heal once by any of the methods mentioned. Here alpha tocopherol treatment can be effective with or without the aid of pressure bandages, etc. Some of those ulcers we have treated successfully have been huge by any standard, and the results have many times far exceeded our expectations.

It is only fair to state that we have failed in some cases, including some which seemed ideal for this treatment, and that in two cases, I recall, the ulcers were subsequently healed by others. I would like to mention them first since they explain both the chief mode of action of alpha tocopherol treatment and the obvious reason for the initial failure.

One occurred in a man, aged 62, who was treated for six months with some help, but whose treatment seemed doomed to failure. He was sent to a surgeon who inserted needles into the femoral artery and injected pure oxygen. The initial reaction was spasm of the artery, with blanching of the limb, and then a suffusion with increased color of the tissues. After two months the ulcers were nearly healed. This man had been a severe diabetic for years, and probably the combination of arteriosclerosis in the arteries of the legs and the varicose veins were the reason that the varicose ulcer would not heal with alpha tocopherol alone.

The second patient was 71 when first seen, and her ulcer has just now healed, nine years later. It was five inches by three inches approximately, when first seen, and responded fairly well at first to alpha tocopherol ointment and alpha tocopherol by mouth. However, after it became about one-quarter healed, further treatment with various adjuvant methods failed to heal it. She was consequently referred to a surgeon, who hospitalized her for months and applied a treatment he had devised and which has apparently been used successfully on other patients. The leg was enclosed in a plastic boot and stocking and pure oxygen piped into the enclosed plastic chamber so formed. The treatment was repeated two or three times over the course of four years, and the ulcer healed completely.

Two comments need to be made. Both patients continued their oral alpha tocopherol, and this may have helped. However, the chief point of interest is that it was increased oxygen supplied to the tissues that led to the healing, and that is precisely what vitamin E does in a different way— namely, by reducing the oxygen need of tissues. However, as has been so often stated in this book, the degree of oxygen conservation varies widely in individual patients.

By contrast, let us consider a case treated in 1949, in which presumably the specific action of oxygen conservation of alpha tocopherol allowed the tissues to heal themselves completely and rapidly. Obviously the degree of oxygen conservation here was maximal. Certainly, everything was against such a result. The patient was very obese, weighing 254 pounds, partly because of inactivity necessitated by the painful legs. She had an initial blood pressure of 228/124, and the ulcers were huge and had been so for 13 years with no signs of healing. Indeed, we initially told her we felt sure we could not help her, but were willing to try if she wished us to.

She had an ulcer on the right leg which almost completely girdled the lower one-third of the leg, while the ulcer on the left leg was equally wide and somewhat larger, extending beyond the natural crease between the foot and ankle into the upper part of the foot.

Since this was in 1949, before the advent of effective antihypertensive drugs, because of the hypertension her initial dose of alpha tocopherol was only 100 units a day. She was given alpha tocopherol ointment to use *only on her left leg*, the worse one, since we wanted to assess the degree of improvement from the ointment alone, especially since so small an oral dosage was probably relatively useless, except as a slow relaxer of the peripheral resistance in her vascular tree and a consequent lowering of blood pressure.

On her second visit it was obvious that there was much greater improvement in her left leg than in the right, and so thereafter the ointment was used on both legs. Her blood pressure did drop to 184/88, but for financial reasons she did not increase her dosage of alpha tocopherol as requested, until her family finally assisted her. On 600 units of alpha tocopherol a day, given after the fall in blood pressure, these huge ulcers healed.

Note that again she demonstrated the type of healing that is so characteristic of vitamin E treatment — in spite of no specific attempts to keep the wound sterile, the infected granulation tissue of the ulcer base cleared up, and healthy granulation tissue replaced the infected tissue, forming an ideal base for the inward growth of the epithelium. There was no contraction or heaping-up of the new skin, and it was nontender.

This was one of several such cases which exhibited a unique characteristic noted first with some disbelief and no ready explanation — self-grafting. As of now, the likely explanation seems to me that the flakes of skin around the ulcer seem to be displaced by the bandaging and to fall upon the healthy granulation tissue of its base. If the cell falls with its deep surface inward, it grows as an island, and such islands, eventually touching other such growing islands or the periphery of the ulcer, coalesce. We have seen several cases, such as this, who partially grafted themselves.

The very first case I saw of a large, chronic, persistent ulcer, healed completely, was one I never did treat, although I have seen the patient almost annually for years because of the concomitant collagenosis.

She lived in a mining town in the Canadian north, had had a persistent large ulcer on the medial side of the lower one-third of her leg in an area of extreme collagenosis and pigmentation. As a result, her foot felt numb all the time. This ulcer was treated with various ointments and compression bandages for years, and finally the patient consulted a second doctor, who pointed out the sentinel vein above the ulcer and sent her south to a university hospital where this vein was surgically ablated. This surgery did not help, and after several months she consulted a third physician who advised hot soaks. This treatment as carried out by the patient proved to be too severe, and the added insult to the already anoxic tissues surrounding the ulcer led to a marked increase in size. She then returned to her original doctor, who was angry with her, apparently, and said that now there was nothing that could be done but amputation.

Just at this time, all Canadian papers carried articles for and against the use of vitamin E for cardiovascular disease. Its use was advocated by our group but immediately condemned by experts, none of whom knew what vitamin E was and none of whom had ever used it or seen a patient on whom it had been used. However, this patient seized upon the hope it offered and began to take it "in large doses" as vaguely recommended in these newspaper reports.

Soon she noticed an increased tingling in her foot; the ulcer began to heal a little, and she tried then to enlist her doctor's interest. He wouldn't see her until she consented to amputation, so she continued to treat herself. After several months, she appeared at my office, related the above history, and showed me a leg with a large healed ulcer scar in an area of collagenosis, involving the lower one-third of the leg with maximum purplish discoloration.

In the 22 years since, the collagenosis first softened and then completely disappeared. We have many cases in which the area of collagenosis decreases and the area seems to soften, but she is still the only one in which it has disappeared. Almost all cases with varicose eczema, and with collagenosis, show a definite and often marked decrease in the pigmentation in the area.

A word of caution: About one patient in ten cannot tolerate full strength alpha tocopherol ointment. Some cannot tolerate it at all, but most of these sensitive persons can tolerate it when it is diluted 50-50 with petroleum jelly—its usual base.

CHAPTER 15. *DIABETES*

DIABETES MELLITUS BY DEFINItion is a disorder of the carbohydrate metabolism. Associated with a disturbance of the normal insulin-producing mechanism, it is characterized by excessive levels of blood sugar (hyperglycemia) and glycosuria, sugar in the urine. Accompanying the diabetic disorder of the carbohydrate metabolism, there are readily demonstrated abnormalities of the protein and fat metabolisms which may give rise to simple acidosis, to ketosis, a type of acidosis involving abnormal production of acetone, to coma, and to death. Diabetics often—but not always—have inherited a predisposition toward the disease, although when it develops late in life in maturity-onset diabetes, its principal cause may well be improper diet. Whether the disease is congenital or contracted, when it reaches its fully developed form, those afflicted by it show weakness, lassitude, and loss of weight. Excessive thirst and frequent urination are prominent symptoms.

Since Banting and Best produced insulin in 1921 and demonstrated its ability to control the level of glucose in the blood and urine, medical treatment has been able to prolong the lives of diabetics by an average of 20 years or more over the previous life expectancies of these unfortunates. The majority of diabetics can look forward to reasonably long and productive lives after their metabolic abnormality is discovered. As medical ability to control blood sugar levels has improved and the armamentarium of available drugs has increased, it has more and more become the case that diabetic patients die, not of diabetes, but of the derivative abnormalities of the cardiovascular system that are either caused by or associated with the diabetic condition.

Beginning with secondary abnormalities of the small blood vessels, and in no way corrected by insulin administration, the condition eventually leads to kidney failure, or blindness, or neuritis, hypertension or congestive heart failure, or a combination of two or more of these problems.

Thus, while in the last 48 years enormous progress has been made in the treatment of diabetes and in the accumulation of far more extensive and precise knowledge of what causes the hyperglycemia and of the variety of ways it may be controlled, little progress has been made in the vascular aspects of the disease. With modern treatment, the control of the blood-sugar levels can be obtained quite consistently. Consequently it is the prevention and treatment of the effects on the vascular system that have become the major problems of diabetes. While some diabetic specialists would disagree, a large number of experts in this disease believe that whether the disease is mild, moderate, or severe and whether control is excellent or poor in no way alters the progress of the vascular damage.

In all diabetics, there is apparent a thickening of the basement membrane of the small arterioles. As this thickening increases, there is intercapillary inflammation in the kidneys (glomerulonephritis) which results. Eventually large masses of transparent (hyaline) material appear, followed by hardening and destruction of the glomeruli.

These same changes occur in the vessels of skin, nerves, muscles, and various other organs. The retinal changes involve also small aneurysmal dilatations of the venules or venous ends of the capillaries. These may rupture and lead to vascularization of the vitreous humor with scarring and retinal detachment. Premature atherosclerosis frequently involves most of the large vessels, especially the cerebral, coronary, and peripheral vessels, particularly of the legs. As well as the usual type of atherosclerosis, Monckeberg's sclerosis is also increased, and there may be premature calcification of these large and intermediate arteries as a result.

It is well to point out that diabetes is a relatively common disease affecting just under two per cent of the population, although in the age group over 60 as many as ten per cent may be affected. Some drugs interfere with carbohydrate metabolism, and so do certain hormones, such as the adrenal corticosteroids and pituitary growth hormone and the chlorothiazides. Of course, surgery to the pancreas by ablation of the islet cells or inflammatory disease can cause the disease.

Since the advent of insulin and the antibiotics, deaths from coma have become relatively rare, while deaths from cardiovascular disease have more than tripled.

Our involvement with diabetes mellitus and its vascular complication began early. Since alpha tocopherol had proven so effective in our original cardiac cases and since there was so very little that doctors could do with such cases, we innocently expected quick confirmation and rapid general adoption of this treatment. When the great local authorities, none of whom knew what alpha tocopherol was (none of whom had ever used it in a single case, or had seen a single case in whom it had been used) stated for publication that the drug was useless, we turned to the treatment of cases of peripheral vascular disease where the condition before treatment could be seen visually; could be photographed before, during, and after treatment, and in which, therefore, the results were irrefutable. Among such cases treated were many with gangrene of extremities, with perforating ulcers, etc., due to their diabetes. Involvement with these cases, of course, meant total involvement in the patients' care, and other aspects of their response were perforce noted.

Now we can confidently state that every diabetic must have adequate control of his disease through diet and insulin or another anti-diabetic drug so that he will not develop coma or hyperglycemia reactions. It is of equal importance that he have alpha tocopherol to minimize the result of his vascular involvement. All three are indispensable for effective treatment.

There has been very substantial support for the use of alpha tocopherol in diabetes mellitus, probably because the outlook in diabetic arteritis is so hopeless without it, and the results with it are so rapid, so obvious, and so good (42) (44) (50) (51) (52) (53) (54) (55) (56) (57) (69).

We have had so many cases of gangrene of the extremities, in which only the tissue already dead when treatment started was lost, that it is hard to choose case histories. Reproductions in color of two such cases can be found in the *Canadian Medical Association Journal* (76, No. 9, May 1, 1957, p. 730).

A woman aged 85, developed gangrene of the left great toe. When she was seen in consultation with her physician, the gangrene had extended primally to the level of the web between the great toe and the second toe. She had just been diagnosed as a diabetic, with this lesion the first indication. Her blood pressure was 150/92.

She was given 600 units of alpha tocopherol daily, in addition to control of her diabetes with an 1,800-calorie diabetic diet and 58 units of insulin. She was not hospitalized. Poor local hygiene led to infection, which spread proximally to about the level of the metatarsophalangeal joint. At this point, four days after treatment began, the dosage of alpha tocopherol was doubled. The live tissue just proximal to the gangrenous tissue became reddened, and a line of demarcation formed and separated the living from the dead tissue. One month later the dead toe was cut away. With the loss of the gangrenous tissue, the insulin requirement dropped to 15 units a day.

By the end of four months, the wound left after amputation had healed completely.

The following case is of interest, because it has been so positively stated in several textbooks and medical journals that diabetic gangrene involving the heel cannot be conservatively treated, but means that above-the-knee amputation must be done.

A woman, aged 61, was brought to the Shute Institute with gangrene involving the heel of the right foot. It had begun as a small ulcer some ten months previously. She had been a known diabetic for 33 years and had been well controlled for all those years.

On examination, her blood pressure was 165/85. Her urine showed no glucose although her fasting blood sugar was 280 mg. per cent. She was very thin and seemed almost comatose, though slowly obeying orders from her daughter and the doctors. I remember that we told the daughter that we thought the condition too advanced, but would try to help. Within seven days there was a definite line of demarcation forming between the living and the dead tissue as if a knife had been used. On 1,200 units of alpha tocopherol daily her insulin requirement dropped from 35 to ten units daily. By the end of four and one-half months the gangrenous heel pad had been nearly completely separated by the proliferation of capillary buds and the necrosis of the dead cells immediately adjacent. The gangrenous tissue extended to the periosteum of the bone beneath and entirely through the subcutaneous tissue in its center so as to expose muscle fibers.

Here occurred the unique and most valuable characteristic of the healing of wounds under alpha tocopherol treatment, confirmed elsewhere (89). The epithelial tissue healed without contracture, and so the healed wound showed no shrinking and no tenderness, and she was able to walk in perfect comfort on a rubber pad in her shoe. Her insulin requirement was stabilized at ten units daily.

In our book *Alpha Tocopherol (Vitamin E) in Cardiovascular Disease*—now long out of print—are color pictures of a large perforating ulcer in a diabetic, healed with alpha tocopherol.

Two cases of relatively successful treatment of the retinal changes in diabetes mellitus are worth reporting. However, in our experience, treating the effects of vascular changes in the brain and retina is much less satisfactory than treating the relatively similar abnormalities in heart, kidney, and extremity. This is to be expected, since nerve cells are so highly specialized and so extremely sensitive to anoxia.

Whereas the heart functions as a whole pump and can work efficiently with a large area knocked out by disease, as is so often the case after recovery from a massive infarction, the brain works as a myriad of independent cells, each with its special and prescribed function. Therefore, we do not like to treat the victims of cerebral accidents, especially when we see them first some weeks or months after the initial accident. Though we can often return to normal function the oxygen-lacking but still-living areas around the area of softening, the total result is moderate help only. To take a bed patient out of bed, to make a chair patient able to walk with a cane, to make a patient who can walk with a cane walk without one are relatively hollow victories, in comparison with the results of alpha tocopherol treatment of cardiac cases.

The same principle applies to diabetic patients losing their sight. With alpha tocopherol, the process can be slowed or halted in many and reversed to a moderate degree in some few; but on the whole results are not very good.

I first saw one man, aged 47, on November 5, 1959. He had been a diabetic for 27 years. Five years previously he had suffered a retinal hemorrhage in his right eye which left him with ten per cent vision. He had four separate hemorrhages in the left eye in the previous two years, the last one three weeks before I saw him. He had no other complaints. On 800 units of alpha tocopherol, both eyes showed improvement, and within six weeks he was able to drive his car. The right eye, in which he was nearly blind, definitely improved.

His diabetic specialist on September 21, 1960, stated that there had been a remarkable change, that the hemorrhages in both eyes were becoming absorbed and were clearing up, although there was very little subjective change. His ophthalmologist became very excited on examining his eyes and said he had never seen anything such as this before.

On November 1, 1960 this patient fell 28 feet, broke four ribs, and suffered facial injuries and an external hemorrhage of the left eye, but no retinal damage. The right eye had continued to clear, and vision was improving.

By September 1, 1961, his diabetic specialist said that he could see through the old hemorrhage in the vitreous and could see the retina for the first time in two years. His field of vision in this eye was definitely expanding.

Improvement continued slowly until June of 1966 when he developed a small hole in the retina. However, his ophthalmologist told him not to let anyone touch it. "Whatever you're doing, keep it up," he said. The regression of the scar tissue in the retina was remarkable, he had never seen better, and there were no signs of fresh hemorrhages. Two months later the hole was seen to be sealing itself off.

In February of 1968 he reported continued improvement in the right eye, but he had just had a fresh hemorrhage in the left, the first in nearly nine years. By November of 1968 his eyesight was about the same as when I first saw him in November of 1959.

The second patient was 35 when first seen on September 30, 1958. He had been a diabetic for 20 years. His eyesight was deteriorating, and he had had hemorrhages in both eyes for the past six years. His left eye was nearly blind. He showed other evidence of arteriosclerosis and had a three-plus albuminuria, for example.

On 600 units of alpha tocopherol a day, his eyesight began to improve within six weeks and was nearly normal in six months. His albuminuria was greatly decreased, and he was feeling really well.

In June of 1962 he suffered a fresh hemorrhage in one eye, and his dosage of alpha tocopherol was promptly doubled. His eyesight returned to normal within two weeks. He admitted that he had become careless and had decreased his alpha tocopherol to 400 units a day.

On April 18, 1963 he suffered an anterior myocardial infarction, this in spite of 1,000 units a day of alpha tocopherol. While in the hospital, he read for many hours a day, and among his books was one on very poor, cheap yellow stock with relatively poor type. With armchair treatment and an increase in his vitamin E, he made an uneventful recovery. As of the present, he takes 48 units of insulin a day. He owns a dry cleaning plant but moonlights as a maintenance engineer in a large hospital-heating plant. He has a two-plus albuminuria. He sees and reads well obviously, since both of his occupations require that he be able to do so.

It is now nearly 11 years since he was first treated with alpha tocopherol. It should be remembered that many other physicians, including ophthalmologists have also had very good results (55) (58) (107).

CHAPTER 16. *KIDNEY DISEASE*

THE TERM "GLOMERULONE-phritis" is used to designate a number of acute and chronic diseases of both kidneys which may be inflammatory, but without forming pus or being degenerative. They are characterized by albumin and blood in the urine. In the acute phase, edema, high blood pressure, and nitrogen retention are present. In the terminal phase, these are almost always present.

This disease was first adequately described by Richard Bright in the nineteenth century. He recognized the fact that acute nephritis usually followed an infection.

There has been a definite cause-and-effect relationship established in the majority of cases of acute glomerulonephritis between an infection with Group A hemolytic streptococci, frequently type 12 strain, and the onset of the disease after a latent period of one to four weeks. Many consider the disease an immune reaction to the infection. Infections with streptococcus viridans and pneumococci can also lead to acute glomerulonephritis.

The kidney appears normal in size or slightly enlarged, but is pale with punctate hemorrhages on the surface. Sections under the microscope show the glomeruli, which are coils of blood vessels, swollen, with the lumina or inner passages of the capillaries diffusely narrowed by proliferations of endothelial cells. Usually, polymorphonuclear leucocytes are present in the lumina of the capillaries and, occasionally, appear to completely close them off. At times, tissue death of some capillary loops, due to thrombi, can be seen, often with adhesions to Bowman's capsule.

There are also deposits of the clotting agent fibrin, commonly concentrated in Bowman's space. As a result, with healing, small areas of scarring develop. In the early stages there is a moderate to severe interstitial edema and, later, interstitial fibrosis.

The chronic phase shows diffuse involvement of all glomeruli by endothelial hypercellularity. As the disease progresses, there are obliterated and scarred glomeruli, adhesions, and hyalinization.

The disease affects people of all ages, but it occurs in males twice as frequently as females. Classical symptoms are bloody urine, a reduced quantity of urine, puffiness around the eyes, and edema of feet or ankles.

Headache, malaise, loss of appetite, with often some aching in the lumbar region, are common symptoms. In mild cases, there may be no signs or symptoms other than edema and moderate hypertension, whereas in severe cases, massive edema, dyspnea, nausea and vomiting, convulsions or coma, extreme hypertension, and enlarged heart, with gallop rhythm, may be present along with such other signs of circulatory congestion as visual disturbances with papilledema and retinal hemorrhages. Conversely, gross hematuria and edema may be the only manifestations, and even these signs may be absent. Many cases are discovered only because the patient was given a routine urinalysis.

This latter aspect of the disease explains why accurate statistics are virtually nonexistent. Certainly, less than five per cent die in hospital in the acute phase. Of the 95 per cent who leave the hospital, some go on to the chronic phase, while others become apparently healed. Many live for 20 to 30 years or more with no clinical evidence except slight albuminuria and slight hematuria. In many of these, kidney function slowly decreases, although symptoms do not appear until the function has become less than 20 per cent. Then nocturia, elevated blood urea nitrogen, anemia, and hypertension develop.

In using vitamin E in the treatment of impaired kidney function and in the treatment of noneclamptic pregnancy toxemia it was occasionally observed that albuminurias and edemas either disappeared or were much improved. These experiences, together with the prior work of Martin and Moore—who found that the kidneys of chronically E-deficient rats revealed extensive degeneration of the renal convoluted tubules, the loops of Henle, and the collecting tubules—suggested that it might prove to be of value to treat patients with acute nephritis by means of vitamin E.

Alpha tocopherol has a direct effect upon capillary permeability, reducing the abnormal capillary permeability that is present with most injurious agents. It therefore, has a direct effect upon the glomerular capillaries, which reduces the local edema both in the glomeruli and the interstitial tissues. It does this within hours and protects against any tendency toward necrosis of capillary loops. It prevents or removes the thrombi associated with the pathological process. Excellent results are obtained by its administration early in the disease, the earlier the better.

There are very few conditions in which the result of treatment is so rapid and so complete as a case of acute glomerulonephritis treated as soon as the diagnosis has been established. Of course, when the patient is seen later in the development of the disease, after necrosis of some of the glomeruli, with scarring and scar-tissue contraction, alpha tocopherol can be of great use, but only through the restoration of function and normalcy to those glomeruli still surviving.

The decrease of oxygen-need, characteristic of the action of the drug, allows the tissues to combat the injury better and is an important factor in establishing maximum recovery.

Again we call attention to the extensive confirmation of the excellent results with this treatment by other physicians (17) (82) (83) for example.

A girl, aged 14 years, was first seen on March 3, 1946. A history of one attack of acute glomerulonephritis at five years was elicited. There had been several subsequent upper respiratory tract infections, none of which had presented any urinary complications. Physical examination then revealed an acute follicular tonsillitis, a purulent nasal discharge and acute right-sided otitis media, moderate edema of the face, eyelids, hands, and ankles, and a fever of 103 degrees. Three days later, on March 6, a gross hematuria and four-plus albuminuria appeared.

The treatment begun on March 7, 1946, consisted of bed rest, a rigid "nephritic diet" which excluded salt, milk, and meat, as well as a daily dose of 200 units of vitamin E. By March 9 her temperature had fallen to normal, and her edema had disappeared. By March 21 all gross hematuria had ceased. By March 26 there was no longer any microscopic hematuria, and the albumin in the urine had decreased to a mere trace. It is interesting to note that no casts were found throughout the period of treatment, despite careful microscopic search for them.

During a routine examination on September 3, 1946, an upper respiratory tract infection was revealed, this time in the form of a subacute pharyngitis with a temperature of 99 degrees. There was also microscopic hematuria again, but no albuminuria. She had not received any vitamin E since the end of the preceding March. It was at once administered as before. In 48 hours all microscopic hematuria had disappeared. Weekly observations since have shown no albuminuria, no casts, no white or red cells. She has started to grow rapidly, and her family state that she is feeling better than she has for years.

Another early case was that of a boy, four years of age. On August 18, 1946, this patient developed acute tonsillitis, with a fever of 102.3 degrees. There was also oliguria and frequent vomiting, but no abdominal or costovertebral tenderness. He was treated with the classical dosage of sulfamerazine, and his temperature reverted to normal in 36 hours. On August 26 he passed normal appearing urine in the morning, but at 1:00 p.m. his urine was "as red as beet juice," and when this was examined it revealed a tremendous hematuria and three-plus albuminuria. The boy was immediately given a daily dose of 150 units of vitamin E. Twenty-four hours later his urine had become grossly clear of blood. In 48 hours from the onset of his hematuria there was no albumin in it, nor could any red blood cells be found microscopically. On September 3 his tonsils were still swollen but not inflamed, and the boy's urine again showed no albumin and only two red and one white cell per low power field. A urinalysis on September 15 showed no cells. He has been perfectly well since.

Male, aged 16 years. This boy suffered from a chronic abscess of his left lower first molar which developed early in June, 1946. On August 9, 1946, while on a fishing trip on Manitoulin Island, he developed a sore throat with malaise, nausea, and vomiting and, on one occasion, a chill. His face began to swell on August 11, and by the morning of August 12 his ankles and fingers were also swollen considerably. This edema gradually progressed. When he was first seen by the writer on August 16 his eyes were nearly closed, and the outline of his ankle bones could not be seen. His urine at that time showed a three-plus albumin, and there were many red and white cells to be seen microscopically. There was no fever at this time, however.

Treatment was started immediately and consisted of bed rest with a daily dose of 300 units of vitamin E. An abscessed tooth was removed at once (August 16), revealing a pus pocket extending deeply into the underlying alveolar bone.

By August 18 the microscopic hematuria had decreased, and only a trace of albumin remained. All edema had disappeared. On August 20 no albumin or blood cells were detectable in the urine, and the patient "felt well." He became ambulant on August 23 just seven days after treatment began and returned at once to his work in a garage. An examination on September 3 showed no albuminuria or edema and only two to three erythrocytes per low power field in his urine. He had continued to work and feel well. Curiously, his friends comment that his "face is not as fat" as it has been for at least four years past. An examination on October 10, 1946, showed no microscopic cellular elements or albuminuria.

A ten-year-old girl was brought to me at the urging of a

local osteopath whose vacation cottage adjoined that of her parents. While at the cottage the child had developed a severe upper respiratory tract infection, which was followed by some edema and led to the diagnosis of acute nephritis by her family physician. She was referred to the largest and most prestigious children's hospital in Canada where she spent some weeks without resolution of her nephritis. Her infection left her with a chronic antrum infection. She was returned to her home under the care of her family physician, and I saw her approximately 11 months later. She had gross edema of ankles, legs, lower back, and abdomen and of her eyelids. She had a four-plus albuminuria, numerous casts, and a few red cells and leucocytes per high power field.

She was given 300 units of alpha tocopherol a day. In two weeks all the edema had cleared up, but she still showed a one-plus albuminuria. She was well enough to go to school, although she twice showed a slight increase in albuminuria with an acute upper respiratory tract infection. She continued to have a trace of albuminuria and so was returned to the children's hospital for evaluation. Now they decided that they could safely do a "radical antrum" operation, and following this she lost all clinical and laboratory signs of her nephritis.

A postscript should here be added. She was ten years old when first seen in 1948. Ten years later she was accepted in this same children's hospital as a nurse-in-training. During her training she was assigned to a ward with a large number of nephritics getting no effective treatment that she could see. She was greatly disturbed by this, since she knew how rapidly and well they would respond to proper treatment. She took her problem home with her to the osteopath who had sent her to me. Of course, his advice was that as a nurse-in-training she must remain helpless to do anything for these children.

If and when she graduated she could decide for herself what course she should take and whom she should approach. It is sad when the treatment available is so nearly nothing when adequate treatment is available and when doctors in charge must know that it is.

This again is a major reason for this book. It reminds me so much of the treatment given my uncle who died and my two brothers who very nearly died of lobar pneumonia in the days before the sulfa drugs and antibiotics were available, and the contrast between their experience and the occasional patient with a similar pneumonia who is now so easily and so successfully treated.

A red-headed boy 14 years old was admitted to hospital on June 6, 1952, two days before we saw him. He had been treated by a pediatrician and carefully investigated before we were called in to supervise his treatment. His illness had begun two weeks before admission with a sore throat, fever, and cough. He had noted a "stomach-ache" and slight headache the day before admission, accompanied by a darkening of his urine. His ankles and legs had begun to swell on the day of admission.

On examination, his eyelids and cheeks appeared to be puffy. The retinae were edematous. A systolic murmur was heard, loudest in the mitral area and transmitted to the axilla. Breath sounds were diminished in the right base. He showed marked pitting edema about the ankles and feet, the edema extending to the knees. His blood pressure was 194/126. His urine showed no sugar, a two-plus albuminuria, three to six leucocytes, and 25 to 40 red cells per high power field. His N.P.N. was 29.6 mgm. per cent, creatinine 1.1 mgm. per cent, and cholesterol 248 mgm. per cent. His hemoglobin was red blood cells 4,030,000 and white blood cells 7,900. An X-ray of the chest taken three days after admission and 12 hours after his first dose of alpha tocopherol showed enlargement of the heart, pulmonary congestion, and a small right-sided pleural effusion.

Alpha tocopherol was given on the third evening after admission (on June 8th at 6 p.m.), and thereafter, during his hospital stay he was given 450 international units daily. His progress is best indicated by the following table:

Date	Blood Pressure	Albuminuria	W.B.C. in Urine	R.B.C. in Urine	Edema
June 6	194/126	2 plus	3-6	25-50	2 plus
June 7	174/110	2 plus	4-8	50-75	2 plus
June 8	174/112	2 plus	3-5	100-200	2 plus
June 9	186/120	trace	occ.	100-150	2 plus
June 10	180/120	1 plus	15-25	150-200	1 plus
June 11	168/116	1 plus	1-2	50-75	trace
June 12	142/102	1 plus	10-15	occ.	0
June 13	138/98	1 plus	5-10	3-5	0
June 14	126/92	1 plus	20-25	occ.	0
June 15	130/90	3 plus	5-10	25-50	0
June 16	122/90	1 plus	3-5	25-50	0
June 17	130/90	Not done			
June 18	130/90	0	0	occ.	0
June 19	130/90	Not done			
June 20	130/90	0	0	0	0
June 24	120/80	0	0	0	0
July 8	120/80	0	0	0	0
Aug. 11	115/70	0	0	0	0

His temperature reached a daily high of 99.3 degrees until June 9, dropped to normal until June 14 when it reached 101.3 degrees; but with continued alpha tocopherol therapy and nothing else, it was normal on June 15 and subsequently. Note that following this exacerbation of fever he had a transient increase in red cells in his urine.

He was discharged 12 days after we saw him first, clinically well. An X-ray of the chest on June 19 showed a return of the heart to normal size and shape and complete resolution of the effusion, although there was still some pulmonary congestion.

He has been perfectly well since. There is now no cardiac murmur.

Another patient was a red-headed boy aged six years. In January, 1953 he had "flu" twice and following his second attack developed hematuria, almost daily headache, severe nausea and vomiting, and fever. He was hospitalized on February 6, 1953 and placed under the care of a pediatrician who investigated the case thoroughly before arriving at the diagnosis of acute nephritis. Blood agglutinations, tuberculin tests, blood cultures, blood chemistry — all these tests were essentially negative. His hemoglobin was 49 per cent. His red cell count was 2.5 million and his sedimentation rate 20 mm. per hour. The urinalysis revealed a trace of albumin and three to six red cells per high power field. His temperature reached 100 degrees on admission to hospital, and he ran a daily fever thereafter until February 21. His treatment before he was placed in our hands on February 23, 1953 was conservative. He was given only a "meat-free and egg-free diet." On February 12 he was transfused with whole blood because of his anemia, and on February 16 he was given a normal diet. On February 18 he was given aureomycin for one day only.

The sequence of his urinalysis is shown in the following table:

Date	Albuminuria	White Cells per h.p.f.	Red Blood Cells
February 6	trace	3-6	3-6
February 7	trace	3-5	5-10
February 8	2 plus	3-6	50-75
February 9	2 plus	10-15	3-5
February 10	3 plus	10-15	100-150
February 11	2 plus	25-50	3-5
February 12	4 plus	0	10-15
February 13	Not done		
February 14	4 plus	3-5	200 plus
February 15	4 plus	25-50	100-150
February 16	4 plus	3-5	10-15
February 17	4 plus	5-10	75-100
February 18	2 plus	3-5	25-50
February 19	2 plus	5-10	75-100
February 20	1 plus	3-5	25-50
February 21	1 plus	occ.	75-100
February 24	trace	3-5	10-15
February 26	0	2	0

Physical examination on admission revealed pallor, no obvious throat infection, a palpable spleen, no edema. An X-ray on February 7, 1953 "showed spleen down a slight distance below left rib margin. There is an increase in the transverse diameter of the heart, which appears fairly marked, and some increase in the bronchovascular markings in both hilar regions."

On February 23, 1953 another X-ray revealed: "residual pulmonary congestion left upper and right lower lobes. No other abnormality in the heart and lungs. Heart shadow now normal."

As has been indicated, we began to treat him on February 23, 1953. We ordered no change in treatment *except* the addition of 400 international units of alpha tocopherol daily. Within three days his urine cleared up completely, and it has remained normal since.

Still another case was a boy, aged four years, who was seen first at the age of 22 months for congenital heart disease. He was one of those sent to Dr. Gordon Murray in Toronto for investigation, although he was asymptomatic on alpha tocopherol therapy. Dr. Murray agreed that he had either an interauricular or interventricular septal defect, and we agreed that he should be investigated still further when older. Late in May, 1952, he developed hematuria two weeks after an attack of flu. He had had no alpha tocopherol for some time before this because of financial difficulties due to his father's illness. He was, of course, once more immediately given 300 international units of alpha tocopherol daily. His urine was virtually free of red cells and albumin in three days and was perfectly normal in one week. He has remained well since.

A girl patient was 14 years old when first seen on August 18, 1966, with a history of glomerulonephritis since the age of four, with a mild fever every afternoon since. At the age of five a pyleogram and catheterization confirmed the diagnosis. At age 13, she had an episode of difficulty in voiding with some burning and pain and pyuria.

On 800 units of alpha tocopherol daily, she still ran a slight but decreased fever for six weeks, since when it has remained normal.

There is no evidence on urinalysis of red cells, white cells, or casts, and she has no urinary symptoms.

However, the greatest change is in the patient herself. She feels completely well, and her mother confirms the obvious and great improvement.

An adult male patient was first seen on March 20, 1953, after 27 months in the Veteran's Hospital.

In December, 1945, while in the army, he was hospitalized for 30 days with an attack of acute glomerulonephritis. In March of 1952 he developed ascites (excess fluid in the abdominal cavity), pleural effusion and dependent edema. He was sent home with a four-plus albuminuria and told that they could do no more for him.

When first seen at the Shute Institute in London, he had a three-plus albuminuria, numerous fine, granular and hyaline casts, no leucocytes, but five to ten red blood cells per high power field. He had edema of feet and legs and fluid in the abdominal cavity. He was very pale and slightly cyanotic with obvious dyspnea even at rest.

An initial dose of 600 units of alpha tocopherol daily was prescribed, and he was able to return to work in less than one month. He still had some peripheral edema, and his urine showed a trace of albumen, but was otherwise negative. He eventually bought a gas station where he worked up to 14 hours a day.

He has been well now for 16 years after being sent home from the Veteran's Hospital with a very grave prognosis.

CHAPTER 17. *BURNS*

OF COURSE, DOCTORS ARE SKEPTIcal of any panacea, any treatment which works perfectly for many different diseases or pathological conditions. Such skepticism should be well tempered these days, however, by the general acceptance of broad spectrum antibiotics and of ACTH and Cortisone, used in so many apparently diverse and unrelated areas of medicine. When one understands the action of alpha tocopherol, that it is an antioxidant acting on all the body's tissues; that it acts directly on clots, diminishing the risk of embolism or extension of the clot; that it dilates blood vessels, the capillaries at least, and certainly relieves spasm in arteries; that it decreases abnormal capillary permeability and softens some scars; then it is obvious that it must help almost any condition in which all or part of the problem is due to thrombosis or to decreased blood flow and consequent tissue anoxia.

Vitamin E is not a specific drug with limited effect on a specific organ or type of tissue, but affects all parts of the body.

Thus, many patients born with an abundant supply of sweat glands, when being treated with alpha tocopherol may be somewhat inconvenienced by excessive sweating and need a stronger deodorant. Patients all notice that their fingernails and toenails grow more rapidly, as does the hair. Unfortunately, the vitamin seems of no use in preserving the precious adornment in the male with hereditary alopecia.

It acts on the whole animal as shown by decompression endurance studies on rats and by Lambert's experience with its use in racing greyhounds. A lengthy study has gained it full acceptance for conditioning race horses in the top Canadian racing stable, leading to its wide use by all leading stables. Further support for the vitamin's over-all value is offered by the author's experience in its use for conditioning world champion figure skaters and international champion swimmers.

Thus, though it may seem far afield from the heart, I have learned that vitamin E is of maximum use in treating burns, from the small domestic burn, due to contact with a heated iron or a stove burner or scalding steam and water, to the most severe third degree burns. Here the results are more important, because the scars that result from vitamin E treatment are unique and uniformly render unnecessary the usual costly, protracted skin grafting with resultant pain and agony to the patient.

The implications of the results in burns are staggering to the imagination. Among existing problems, industrial burns, napalm burns, burns to firemen, etc., could be much better treated than they are now in even the great medical centers. We do our best, in a pitifully small way, to rescue such patients and treat them properly as the following cases will illustrate.

Our first case was a boy of six who, as well as his brothers and sisters, was delivered by Dr. Evan Shute. When he suffered a second degree burn to the dorsum of the fingers of his left hand from a hot laundry iron, his father called, not to discuss his treatment, but to find out which of the local surgeons should be entrusted with the care and grafting of the burned hand, particularly important in this case because the child was left-handed. Instead, he was treated at home with 300 units of alpha tocopherol by mouth, since this was before there was such a preparation as vitamin E ointment. The result was excellent. There was no infection and no deepening of the damaged tissue, *i.e.*, only the tissue killed by the heat of the iron was lost. Healing was rapid, and the resulting scar did not contract and was never tender. The boy regained completely normal function. He was not hospitalized and needed no skin grafting or other surgery, because there was no injury to the living tissue just below the necrotic tissue, and so no involvement of the tendons or tendon sheaths immediately below.

A much more serious case was that of another boy of six, who was badly scalded by a kettle of boiling water with multiple burns over his neck, torso, back and front, and left thigh. He was in the hospital for ten weeks under the care of a university professor. A skin grafting operation was performed using a four-inch square area from the right abdominal wall. None of the grafting was successful, and the whole area became grossly infected. The effect on the child was rather frightful. There were large raw areas, and the frequent dressings, along with the excoriated skin from the pus escaping and running over it, had made him a cringing, unhappy pitiful creature. There was infected, heaped up granulation tissue and no evidence of healing except at the ends of the burn on the thigh; and here the scar seemed to be heaped up and contracted like a keloid or pseudokeloid.

By this time alpha tocopherol ointment was available and, alternating with an antibiotic ointment, was used directly on the wound. He was also given 300 units of alpha tocopherol a day by mouth. The infection cleared up in the first four days; and after ten days of treatment, only the vitamin E ointment was used. Complete healing occurred in 13 weeks.

As everyone knows, skin will not grow over heaped up vascular granulation tissue, and we planned to have any necessary skin grafting done when the right time arrived. However, every time we saw him the skin had grown in still further. The heaped up granulation tissue subsided in front of it. Ultimately we found he did not need grafting. Here again the unique characteristics of scars formed under alpha tocopherol therapy were evident. Whereas the scar formed on the thigh when he was first seen was heaped up and seemed to be keloid, the scar formed with alpha tocopherol was smooth and nontender. Moreover, there was no scar tissue contraction. *The areas of healed scar were exactly the same size as the open wounds were when he was first seen.*

In this patient we noted a direct confirmation of the capillary effect of alpha tocopherol. Whenever the ointment was applied, the granulation tissue became swollen and protruded. Therefore, raised well above the former surface of the wound and clearly visible in the swollen tissue, there could be seen numerous dilated capillary buds. If the ointment was carefully removed, the tissues would shrink, would blanch out, and return to the same level as before. This was repeated several times for the education of various doctors, as well as our own investigation, and we have several excellent color slides of this phenomenon.

Five years ago, a man aged 45 decided to retar the roof of his house during his holiday. He heated the tar in a pail on the roof and was almost ready to begin work. When he went to reach for the brush, it fell into the pail. Without thinking, he automatically reached for the brush to rescue it and plunged his hand into the hot tar.

In the office, we used alpha tocopherol ointment on the hand and patiently wiped off the softened tar until the hand was fairly clean. The ointment was applied daily. However, he was unable to return to work for six weeks, since he works in oil and grease all day as an automobile mechanic.

Since recovery, the hand has been normal in every way. There has been no loss of function and no tenderness of tissue, even while he does his heavy work on cars.

Today, his wife told me that when he gets his hand really clean on week-ends, the skin on that hand looks pink like a baby's. There is no scarring evident, and only those who know about the burn would notice it.

Our most recent case was that of a very obese woman aged 58, who was severely burned with boiling water on May 18, 1969. She was at a summer cottage on a cold weekend, getting the cottage ready for the summer. There was a large kettle of water on the wood stove, and her husband thought it was just warm. Not realizing that it was boiling, he poured the whole kettle into a big plastic jug and put it in the bed beside his wife who had lain down to rest. She felt it was hot and looked up at it. With the movement, the top blew off, and the water poured over her. She had on three sweaters and slacks, which held the scalding water to her. She jumped up and ran screaming around the cabin. She had to be taken two miles by boat and 32 miles by road to get to the nearest hospital, from which she was transferred to a large metropolitan hospital for further care.

She had a third degree burn of the left arm from the middle of the arm, involving about two-thirds of the circumference and all of the forearm to the wrist, with all the posterior surface and a half or more of the anterior surface involved. Roughly, the area involved measured 18 inches by eight inches. She involuntarily grasped the left arm with the right hand and sustained a burn on the tips of all the fingers and thumb and a burn on the anterior surface of the wrist from the hypothenar eminence across the crease between palm and forearm and into the thumb.

There was a large burned area under her left breast where the band of her brassiere held the water to her body, and this was 12 inches long and three inches wide at its lateral end.

She had a large burned area involving her "adipose apron," measuring 12 inches by two and one-half inches to four inches, and an area on the anterior abdominal wall extending upwards and inwards for four inches, which was three inches wide. Above, at a right angle to it, there was another area four inches by two and one-half inches.

The crease in her groin was covered by the adipose apron, but immediately below on her left anterior thigh was an area seven inches by two and one-half inches to three inches of scalded area.

When she was able to remove her sweaters at the cottage, the skin of the top surface of her arm and forearm and the bottom surface of the forearm came away in sheets.

She was treated with saline soaks in hospital, and it was explained to her that she would need extensive grafting, that the burns on her left arm were third degree burns, and that most of the rest of her burns were second and third degree. Meanwhile, while she was being prepared for surgery, the burns on the abdomen and under her breast became infected, and pus and blood ran down her body when she stood up, she says now "down her legs as far as her slippers."

She was in agony and says she screamed when they were dressing her wounds and when they were applying the solution which she presumes was with sponges wrung out in saline.

She had been a patient at the Shute Institute years before, and her husband had been my patient, so she signed herself out of the hospital and came to my office. It took a nurse three solid hours to remove the bandages. The area under the breast was covered by thick black crusts from under the edges of which pus flowed. The burns on the left arm presented a raw red area oozing serum and blood. The wounds were then dressed with alpha tocopherol ointment on gauze using an entire one-half pound jar of ointment that first time.

Since it was impossible to get a bed at this time in the local hospital, she went to her daughter's home and the Victorian Order of Nurses, a very capable order of visiting nurses, dressed the wounds daily. The infected areas cleared up in four or five days, and healing began.

Now, three months later, all areas are healed except on the posterior surface of the left arm, which still must be dressed daily, since there are five or six areas about one-quarter to one-half inch across that are open and raw. However, she has been back at work for a couple of weeks as a switchboard operator.

She volunteered the information that as the burns were healing the surfaces were red and angry looking and raised above the surface of the skin, but that as the skin grew in and the area healed, this subsided.

Now the healed areas are still red, but are fading. At the edges for some distance — up to one or two inches in some cases — one must look carefully to see where the burn had been. The burned area on the arm is still elevated above the surrounding tissue.

Again, the unique characteristics of the burn scar healed

under this treatment are very obvious. There is no contraction of scar tissue anywhere, and the scar is already pliable and nontender. She has used 27 pounds of ointment to date. The nurses of the Victorian Order are not only converts, but the most ardent of advocates.

Obviously, anyone familiar with the results of the use of alpha tocopherol for burns must realize the import of such cases. The prevention of shock, of infection, and of toxic injury to the still viable but insulted tissues beneath are specific answers to the major dangers of burns, recognized and poorly combated in every severely burned case in every major hospital and medical center everywhere.

The freeing of hospital beds is of major importance these days, as everyone knows, but the economic consideration is as nothing compared to the elimination of the need of skin grafting in most cases. The agony of the patient with the usual "accepted" methods of treatment is something else to consider. This was the one major feature of this last case which the patient and her husband kept talking about!

CHAPTER 18. *VITAMIN E OINTMENT*

WE FIRST USED ALPHA TOCOPHerol in ointment form for indolent ulcers in 1947, but did not report its use for superficial wounds until the next year.

The oral administration of alpha tocopherol should be begun simultaneously with the topical ointment, since, while either alone may be effective, one complements the other. Open wounds so handled, whether traumatic or ascribable to prolonged decubitus, heal faster, with less scar-tissue contraction, with a more pliable subcutaneous layer and with less tender surface covering, than do such wounds treated in any other way. The usefulness of alpha tocopherol ointment in burns, whether thermal in origin or due to X-ray or radium, has also been demonstrated. Noteworthy is the limitation of necrosis so achieved in thermal burns and this even in severe cases. Prompt application is essential, of course. First-degree burns so treated may almost disappear in two or three days. As we have pointed out elsewhere, there is a singular freedom from infection, toxemia, and contracture which often makes skin-grafting unnecessary. Incidentally, this ointment is excellent for small domestic burns and has a very practical application in the inconvenient, uncomfortable, and very common sunburn.

Elsewhere we have reported the ability of oral alpha tocopherol to improve the circulation in limbs showing small areas of gangrene. By its means the viable tissues just proximal to the dead cells can, by the usual process of capillary budding and phagocytosis of dead cells with liquefaction, separate necrotic from living tissue at the zone of separation. Healing of the raw subgangrenous areas left when the gangrenous patches detach themselves can be accelerated by the local use of tocopherol ointment.

Recalling the early studies of Steinberg, lumbago was early treated by us with inunction of tocopherol ointment over the affected area, followed by heat. Within an hour or so pain and disability could disappear. We have used this treatment on many cases of fibrositis and myositis. The discovery that alpha tocopherol in ointment form apparently penetrated intact skin, and might have a direct effect upon underlying joints, led to trials of this agent on a variety of conditions where diminished blood supply or decreased tissue oxygenation could be a part of the picture. Thus we have seen a few cases of rheumatoid arthritis in which the swelling and pain in the joints were materially reduced and mobility increased. One such patient who had been nearly immobile for 18 months returned to normal activity with residual flexion deformity in but three joints. The ointment, rubbed into fingers showing rheumatoid arthritis, can be especially helpful. Not all cases respond, of course, and our experience is relatively limited.

The ointment is of real value in relieving the itching of the abdominal skin associated so often with striae gravidarum and for pruritus ani or vulvae and even for the irritation of keloids.

A field in which our experience has been extensive is that of chest pain of non-cardiac origin. So often in right-handed persons there is pain in the left chest wall, most frequently found in the fourth or fifth interspace, accompanied by tenderness on pressure between the ribs which may extend around to a point just lateral to the spinous processes of the vertebral bodies. This pain may closely simulate true angina pectoris, since exertion and any resultant deep breathing may irritate the lesion and evoke the pain. It can usually be differentiated from true angina by the fact that it begins with a change in position on sitting in a too-easy chair or on lying on a too-soft mattress, is tender, and is aggravated by coughing, twisting, or even deep breathing. It is frequently misdiagnosed and can even be labeled status anginosus. The variety of terms applied to this condition is evidence of its interest, e.g., intercostal neuritis, spondylitis, even arthritis of the spine. Vitamin E ointment, gently rubbed in for ten minutes, followed by heat for ten minutes and applied to the paravertebral area only, will relieve the pain in one to three days in many cases. Thiamin chloride, given orally or by injection, is very valuable, of course. We often recommend manipulation and note with interest that a recent report has commented favorably on such treatment.

In 1949 Scardino and Hudson reported the beneficial effect of oral alpha tocopherol on Peyronie's disease. We have seen a few such cases co-incidentally in patients under treatment with vitamin E for cardiac conditions. Some have reported improvement, rarely complete; some have no improvement; none have worsened. In one case we suggested that it might be possible to increase the concentration of alpha tocopherol locally by the use of the ointment and heat. It should be noted that this patient has been ingesting a large dosage of alpha tocopherol daily for three years, the status of the Peyronie's disease remaining the same. Using tocopherol ointment the condition improved greatly in three months.

Finally, we wish to report the use of tocopherol ointment in a case of recurring corneal ulcer, in the hope that this suggestion may be tested further by ophthalmologists. A man has been under our care since June, 1954, for intermittent claudication and accordingly has been given 300 to 1,600 units of alpha tocopherol daily. In May, 1957, while taking 750 units daily, he developed a recurrent corneal ulcer for the sixth time since 1940. Originally, a piece of radium paint from an aircraft instrument had flown into his eye, and the resulting ulceration had been treated by an ophthalmologist for six weeks. Originally, and during the ensuing four attacks, ophthalmic ointments of several types and oral and parenteral antibiotics had failed to heal the ulcer until it was cauterized. When this sixth recurrence was noted, we decided to instill half-strength tocopherol ointment. Two days later full strength ointment was applied. The lesion healed in two weeks, and there were no untoward effects from the introduction of the ointment into the eye. No previous observation of this sort has been found in the literature. We may add that his sight has not worsened appreciably with this last episode.

We occasionally see an indolent leg ulcer in which the ointment increases local irritation or even provokes an id rash. Perhaps a dilute ointment containing 15 international units of alpha tocopherol per gram should be used initially on such patients and should be applied on limited areas. If that causes no general or local reaction but does not promote healing in the lesion, then a stronger tocopherol ointment can be used safely.

CHAPTER 19. *TAILORING THE DOSE*

IT IS NOW NEARLY 24 YEARS SINCE we treated the first ten cardiac patients with alpha tocopherol. During these years we have personally cared for or supervised the treatment of more than 30,000 cardiovascular patients. Because much has been learned from this large experience and because of the appearance of some new and useful adjuncts to alpha tocopherol therapy, it now seems a good idea to specify the dosage schedule for the different cardiovascular conditions commonly met in such a practice.

It is noteworthy that time has shown alpha tocopherol to be unique in its ability to prevent coronary thrombosis, to dissolve fresh venous thromboses, and to decrease or abolish the symptoms that usually follow such disasters. Since these symptoms are chiefly limitation of exercise tolerance due to dyspnea, or angina pectoris, or both, the important action of alpha tocopherol here is its oxygen conservation. As shown in the experiments of air-force investigators, the administration of alpha tocopherol to normal animals decreases the oxygen requirements of muscle, cardiac and skeletal. Houchin and Mattill have also demonstrated this action of alpha tocopherol. In cardiac cases the oxygen needs are reduced, so anoxia to the degree that initiates angina pectoris or dsypnea is not reached as readily or at all. It should be noted that there are no safe rival drugs available to contest its powers and usefulness. The other fibrinolysins are still in the cautious, experimental stage.

Although it is about 110 years since Vogel first discovered cholesterol in the aorta, there is still no satisfactory evidence that coronary attacks can be prevented by controlling cholesterol values in the blood stream. Indeed it has been stated that cholesterol is not the major constituent in plaques in the coronary artery, yielding precedence to triglycerides. Talbott's article on cholesterol is refreshingly sane.

The almost universal use of the anticoagulants by cardiologists in treating coronary thrombosis, in both the acute phase and as long-term treatment, followed the paper published in 1948 by Irving S. Wright and his group. Why it took 12 more years for several thousand cardiologists and clinicians to discover that these drugs were of dubious value and also highly dangerous is hard to explain, just as it is hard to explain why these drugs are still in common use in 1969, some nine or ten years after they should have been widely discarded, at least for chronic patients.

Similarly, bed rest for six weeks after an acute coronary episode is apparently more dangerous than useful, as discovered and reported by Samuel Levine in 1952. In this year, 1969, Levine's armchair treatment (with a reduction of the death rate to ten per cent) is just beginning to be used in some parts of Canada by more than the author. As recently as 1964, one great Ontario hospital was reported to be disturbed by its 40 per cent coronary death rate. The conclusion is inescapable that, for 11 years, this hospital had permitted four times as many patients with coronary occlusion to die as in a similar hospital in Boston! Early ambulation was the obvious major difference in the two centers.

Not only is alpha tocopherol the drug of choice in treating coronary artery narrowing and/or occlusion, but it is also effective in treating all other forms of heart disease with or without the help of other old and new drugs, such as digitalis, the chlorothiazides, Rauwolfia, diuretics, and such.

However, as is true for any useful drug, one must know how to use alpha tocopherol and must have a reliable preparation, properly assayed and labeled and one with which the physician is thoroughly familiar. Indeed, general acceptance of alpha tocopherol in treating cardiovascular disease might have been achieved long since had the earliest workers in the field used the same dosage schedule and product that we had used and upon which our original findings were released to the medical profession. For example, *only the alpha fraction* of the tocopherols is really effective. For this reason, it is essential to use a product in which the alpha fraction is assayed. So many of the tocopherol preparations are a combination of the tocopherols, and, unless the alpha fraction is potent and its potency known by assay, one is likely to earn a poor result.

Primarily it is because of its value as fibrinolysin and its oxygen conservation powers that alpha tocopherol is so useful in cardiovascular disease, although in acute rheumatic fever and acute glomerulonephritis its ability to decrease capillary permeability in a very short time may be what allows it to dispel signs and symptoms.

This note is, therefore, intended to serve as a guide to its intelligent therapeutic use. The key to success depends upon fitting the dosage to the individual patient's peculiar requirements. Different forms of cardiovascular disease require different ranges of effective dosage. For example, coronary artery insufficiency, whatever the underlying pathology, responds usually to 800 to 1,200 I.U. of alpha tocopherol daily. However, individual patients may need much more. Starting a victim of chronic rheumatic heart disease on such a dose can lead to rapid deterioration or death. Intermittent claudication may be relieved on 800 I.U. a day, but this rarely. Sixteen hundred I.U. a day seems to be a wiser dose, and 2,400 I.U. can be needed.

Coronary Heart Disease
Angina

(a) Those patients who have a normal blood pressure, *i.e.*, 120/80 or very nearly that, who have angina pectoris on effort or excitement, but no evidence of congestive failure, and whose electrocardiograms do not show evidence of myocardial infarction in the standard or five precordial leads.

These should be checked out very carefully to rule out intercostal tenderness in the left chest, a very frequent finding in right-handed people and a lesion which can simulate angina pectoris due to coronary sclerosis. We treat this intercostal neuralgia intensively in all patients, since it may either complicate a true case of angina pectoris or simulate it in cardiologically normal people.

We give these coronary patients 800 I.U. alpha tocopherol daily for six weeks. Since alpha tocopherol in cardiac patients takes five to ten days to begin to take effect and four to six weeks to diminish or relieve symptoms to the point where the results are obvious to patient and physician alike, we check all such patients after six weeks of treatment and often carry out a practical exercise tolerance test at the end of five or six weeks to establish the approximate degree of improvement.

If all or nearly all symptoms have disappeared, we maintain the patient on that dose indefinitely. He must take the full dose every day, since he can lose all relief from the treatment within three to seven days after cessation of therapy. A diminution of dosage will, of course, lead to a slower but certain return of symptoms. Very rarely a dosage of this degree may lead to gastric distress, but this will nearly always respond to the addition of three teaspoonsful of skim milk powder in a little milk or water after each meal with the added precaution of taking the alpha tocopherol half way through each meal.

If the patient is not improved on the original dosage level we raise it by 200 I.U. per day at six-week intervals until he is relieved or until we must admit defeat. Even then, mindful of our own experience and of Zierler's and Ochsner's work, we maintain a dosage of 800 I.U. a day to prevent intravascular clotting — aware that such patients stand a very real danger of coronary thrombosis.

Formerly we had to be very careful of patients in this category who had an elevated blood pressure, since large doses of alpha tocopherol, by increasing the tone of cardiac muscle, could elevate the blood pressure still more. However, we now start such patients on 800 I.U. a day, and proceed just as above, except that we place them on a suitable dose of hydrochlorothiazide. On their return visit in six weeks the blood pressure is usually lowered and can be satisfactorily controlled. Occasionally, we must add Rauwolfia or other such drugs. Rarely is the blood pressure reading higher than on the original examination.

Coronary Occlusion

(b) Acute phase. The only correct time to begin the treatment of a case of coronary occlusion with alpha tocopherol is immediately upon establishment of the probable diagnosis! In such cases the full value of the oxygen-conserving power of alpha tocopherol and of its ability as a capillary dilator has a chance to salvage the heart. The infarct can be greatly reduced in size, and adjacent tissue death may be largely prevented. Later it is too late to prevent extensive tissue necrosis. Then all that can be done is to promote healing in the damaged myocardium surrounding the infarct, the areas commonly known as the zones of injury and ischemia; to increase the rate and extent of the opening up and establishment of collateral circulation and to ensure a firm scar tissue repair of the infarcted area. Of course, decreasing the oxygen need of the rest of the laboring heart is of real value and usually insures an added chance of survival.

These cases are ideal test problems, since in them all the powers of alpha tocopherol have their chance to demonstrate themselves. Indeed, one of the most dramatic proofs of the value of alpha tocopherol in coronary occlusion is demonstrable here, since in such fresh cases the electrocardiogram will show the change typical of the lesion, but to a diminished degree; thenceforward, the recovery of the electrocardiogram is more rapid and complete than it is without alpha tocopherol. We now have an interesting collection of such electrocardiograms.

The well-known drop in blood pressure that occurs in acute myocardial infarction allows full and immediate dosage in every case. Previously elevated pressures often remain within a normal range after recovery. Some will need antihypertensive drugs later, however.

We now start all acute cases on 1,600 I.U. of alpha tocopherol per day. A smaller dose is certainly adequate in the majority of cases, but it is better to make sure that maximum help is being given.

Postocclusion Status of Coronary Cases

(c) We are seeing more and more fresh occlusions in consultation or in our own practice, but, of course, the majority of post-occlusal cases seen by us during the last twenty years have come weeks, months, or years after their accident. If cardiologists really believe that a majority of patients regain good or near-normal health following an occlusion, they are mistaken. Such patients are not deceived by the usual reassurance and six-monthly visits. The majority of those we have seen have had a definite and usually marked abnormality of the electrocardiogram. In the evaluation of treatment in these patients, the pulse rate and electrocardiographic changes become the best objective evidence of adequate dosage and, therefore, of adequate protection.

Here is one place where the clinician unaccustomed to tocopherol therapy must learn something entirely new. The myocardial infarct itself, the "zone of injury" next to it, and the "zone of ischemia" just outside that again form a total area affecting the electrocardiogram. As time goes on this area either is slightly decreased by the slowly forming anastomoses, or it remains constant, or it gradually spreads as the basic disease process worsens accordingly. The electrocardiogram either shows spontaneous improvement, or reaches a static state for months or years, or gradually shows an increase of abnormality, depending upon whatever variation just described has developed. However, when such a patient responds to adequate alpha tocopherol therapy we believe that the zone of injury may lessen, the zone of ischemia may perhaps become physiologically normal, and the total area can thereby be greatly reduced. At least such improvement is reflected by corresponding changes in the T wave of the electrocardiogram. This sequence, may we repeat, is scarcely known to the older cardiologists because it so rarely occurred in their experience before the day of alpha tocopherol.

For some reason patients with coronary occlusions often respond more rapidly and completely to alpha tocopherol therapy than do those having coronary sclerosis and angina pectoris, but without definite electrocardiographic evidence of infarction. Morris has shown convincingly that coronary thrombosis may be quite independent of atherosclerosis, although angina pectoris presupposes atheromatous changes.

Patients in this category are started also on 800 I.U. a day, with increases of 200 to 400 I.U. a day at six-week intervals, until improvement is obtained.

Rheumatic Heart Disease

(a) *Acute Rheumatic Fever.* The first attack: Here, as with acute coronary occlusion, the proper time to treat the patient is the moment the probable diagnosis is made. Under such circumstances all evidences of disease may disappear in as little as three to seven days — at least by three to four weeks. Fever, joint symptoms and signs, tachycardia, and elevated sedimentation rate will in many a case disappear entirely. Here also, irrespective of age, the full dosage of 600 units daily should be given by mouth.

(b) *Continuing Rheumatic Fever,* with marked damage to the heart, and with or without congestive failure, as long as there is no auricular fibrillation present.

Herein the ideal treatment is still as in (a) above. However, there are many cases in which the damage from earlier attacks is so great that the full dosage cannot be given immediately without precipitating congestive failure. If the heart size is nearly normal and heart damage moderate or relatively slight, we try full dosages as in (a). If we can send the patient to hospital and have full laboratory and other such facilities for treatment, we give a trial of full dosage, since here we are able to detect adverse responses as soon as they occur. In the majority of cases, however, we must treat these patients cautiously, giving 90 I.U. per day for the first four weeks, 120 I.U. daily for the second four weeks, and 150 I.U. for the third four weeks. Usually 150 I.U. is the maximum safe level of dosage.

(c) *Patients with beginning failure, after years of normal or comparatively normal health following recovery from an attack of acute rheumatic fever.*

This group is ideal to demonstrate the value of alpha

tocopherol therapy. Compensation can be restored in most of them within a few weeks, and they seem to continue to improve steadily thereafter. It is in this group that diminution, and even the very occasional disappearance, of murmurs has been demonstrated by Dowd; even diminution of a moderate degree of cardiac enlargement can develop after two to three years of therapy. This is not too hard to understand if one thinks of the properties of alpha tocopherol, especially its effect on scar tissue — and mitral stenosis, of course, is a scar process involving the angles of the cups of the mitral valve.

Many of these patients are first seen early in pregnancy and in these compensation is more difficult to achieve, requiring usually a larger dosage of alpha tocopherol and longer treatment.

Such patients should be started very gradually on alpha tocopherol. It will be 12 to 15 weeks before they notice real improvement. Meanwhile, if they show early congestive failure, it can now be easily and successfully treated with the newer diuretics until the end of this period of three and one-half months, after which such adjuncts to treatment can usually be safely stopped. We start such patients on 90 I.U. a day for one month, then give 120 I.U. for one month and then 150 I.U. permanently. 150 I.U. is usually an effective dose, and there is no need to increase it. Indeed, it may be several years before the maximum safe dose in such cases (300 I.U. a day) can be reached. Any attempt to increase beyond 150 I.U. can precipitate fresh congestive failure or palpitation. Strangely enough, a patient living a normal life on 300 I.U. for years (10 to 15) can sometimes be precipitated into failure by a mere 75 I.U. more.

A few cases require months to show satisfactory improvement, but persistence should turn virtually every case in this category into a satisfied patient.

(d) *Chronic Rheumatic Heart Disease.* These end states show congestive failure, auricular fibrillation, and very little or no exercise tolerance.

These cases which are so very common illustrate the

failure of all conventional methods of treatment in rheumatic heart disease. This stage of partial to complete invalidism lasts for five to ten years, and its effect upon the patient and his relatives is sad to watch.

It is difficult to treat such cases even with alpha tocopherol, because it, of course, requires a miracle to make a heart so badly damaged function well enough to restore the patient even to a limited degree of normal living. A 50 per cent improvement in a patient confined to bed still leaves him an invalid. Yet we have had patients in this category who had spent six to 19 months in bed under classical therapy, who were able to resume full activity and to maintain normal living with increasing strength. This has occurred in as little as a month of tocopherol treatment. Apparently the factors determining the extent of improvement are many and complex, although many of these are obvious to anyone understanding the basic pathology and the pharmacological effect of alpha tocopherol. We could mention just one here — alpha tocopherol has been shown to reduce the oxygen requirement of heart muscle by a great deal.

This type of case is still worth attempting to treat, since the results can be so valuable occasionally. Need we stress the fact that every aid in the pharmacopoeia must be used, especially at first, until the effect of alpha tocopherol has had a chance to show itself? Then gradually these older agents may be dispensed with, or used less often or in smaller dosage.

The most important point in treating these patients is to bring the congestive failure under control as quickly as possible by the use of the right amount of digitalis and diuretics, given as often as is necessary to relieve the failure completely. At the same time alpha tocopherol is begun. If the patient is under *close* supervision he should be given 300 I.U. of alpha tocopherol daily from the beginning, provided the physician is sufficiently experienced in using alpha tocopherol to know when his patient is showing evidence of excessive dosage. Since alpha tocopherol will not show much effect for about ten days and since intensive treatment of the congestive failure should show a steady improvement by the first ten days of treatment, this overdosage is being reached if the patient begins to show signs of increasing failure at about the ten- to 14-day period. If, however, the patient begins to improve more rapidly at this phase, full dosage is maintained thereafter until the fourth week, when the other accessory medications can often be reduced or stopped entirely. Some digitalis, usually much less than before treatment and much less than is necessary during the first two weeks, may be continued. That is a matter for professional experience and judgment.

If however, the patient is one of those who cannot tolerate so large an initial dose, then alpha tocopherol should be stopped for two full days and the slower schedule adopted — 90 I.U. for four weeks, 120 I.U. for four weeks, and then 150 I.U. a day thereafter.

Curiously, patients in this group often do best on 150 I.U. a day — even better, indeed, than on the large dosage. One must find out by trial. For example, one patient was told by a very competent cardiologist that she would never do another bit of work of any kind, but has done her own housework for the last four years, taking 150 I.U. a day and nothing else, except for two short periods — once when she became dyspneic on 180 I.U. a day and once when she reduced her dose to 120 I.U. a day — with the recurrence of complete failure. So narrow a dosage tolerance is fairly common in this type of patient. In no other type is it so necessary to tailor the dose to the individual patient's requirement.

Most of our patients come from many miles away, and so we usually follow the slow dosage procedure. By the end of six weeks on any given dosage one can usually tell if it is the dose that will give the optimum results. Once improvement begins it will usually continue slowly for many months or years. While the improvement is so slow as to be very discouraging for three months or more on this slow schedule, it is really the most accurate way of arriving at the individual's correct dosage.

When too large a dose is given in any type of heart disease, the patient often shows an unusually rapid and encouraging response and then becomes worse again. When this happens, it is evidence that the optimum dosage level was reached and then exceeded. Since alpha tocopherol is rapidly excreted, stop the dosage for three days — no more — and begin again at approximately the right level, or just less.

In tailoring the dose to the individual's requirement, remember the general rule: a patient with a normal or low blood pressure and with no evidence of congestive failure can nearly, but not quite always, tolerate any quantity of alpha tocopherol. "It can do him no harm." So give him enough to do the job. Like digitalis and insulin and thyroid extract, the right dose is the dose that begins to show definite improvement, in four to six weeks in this case. The maintenance dose is the same. However, in the presence of hypertension or congestive failure, in advanced rheumatic heart disease, or both, be careful. Probably you can kill the patient if you are overzealous.

However, an exception to the presence of congestive failure, as a contraindication to high dosage of alpha tocopherol, is coronary heart disease following occlusion. In such a case we give full dosage, and the failure tends to clear up with the disappearance of myocardial anoxia. In rare cases where the patient is obviously dying of congestive failure in hypertensive heart disease the same applies. Tailor your dose to the patient's needs. Maintaining full dosage in the post-occlusive patient maintains better myocardial oxygenation.

Summary

1. Alpha tocopherol has its own mechanics of action on damaged hearts, and its dosage levels, speed of ingestion, rate of excretion, potentialities for harm and toxicity must be understood if it is to be used successfully.

2. There is a dose appropriate to every patient. More or less may harm the patient. It may require weeks or months to determine what his dose should be.

3. Patience and skill are demanded by this type of treatment. There is no simple rule-of-thumb.

CHAPTER 20. *VITAMIN E ON THE MOON*

WHEN THE FIRST MEN TO WALK on the surface of the moon returned to earth, their physical condition was checked with meticulous care. Special attention was paid to medical problems that had developed during previous, shorter flights into space, notably bone demineralization, the development of hemolytic or red cell-destroying anemia, and general weakening of the cardiovascular system evidenced by a highly accelerated pulse rate.

Unlike previous space voyages, the Apollo 11 Moon Walk Crew, Armstrong, Aldrin and Collins, were provided a food supply that had been substantially enriched with vitamin E.

Only preliminary medical information has been released at this writing, and that has appeared in newspapers; but it is noteworthy that there has been no mention at all of the "blood deconditioning process"—a euphemism for hemolytic anemia—that was reported after earlier space voyages of a duration of more than eight days, notably the Borman-Lovell Gemini 7 flight in December, 1965.

Actually, in view of the fact that spacecrafts up to now have carried pure oxygen atmospheres, it is strange that it should have taken so long to recognize the need for vitamin E. It was determined many years ago, at the very beginning of the U.S. program of manned space flights, that crews are better able to withstand the fantastic accelerations required to break free of the earth's gravitational pull in an atmosphere of pure oxygen than in any other type of atmosphere. Yet it is no secret to any scientist that pure oxygen rapidly begins to demonstrate toxic effects. As early as 1935,

Behnke, Johnson, Poppen, and Motley, writing in the *American Journal of Physiology* (110: 565, 1935) showed that pure oxygen is toxic and that as the atmospheric pressure increases, the toxicity of pure oxygen increases also. The hyperbaric administration of oxygen demonstrated toxic effects that quickly became well known; and by 1964 it was possible for a research team writing in *Aerospace Medicine* to assume that the toxic effect of pure oxygen was generally recognized by readers.

This particular paper, titled "Oxygen Toxicity and Vitamin E," was presented by the authors, Drs. Kann, Mengel, Smith, and Horton, at an Aerospace Medical Association meeting in May, 1964. Their paper should have received much wider attention than it did.

At the time their study was performed, it had already been found that when space capsule environments were simulated, with high oxygen concentrations, the volunteers who were subjected to such environments tended to develop convulsions and hemolytic anemia. Kann, Mengel, Smith, and Horton speculated that the toxic effect might derive from the peroxidation of unsaturated fatty acids, a condition that is best prevented in a normal environment by the presence of enough vitamin E in the bloodstream.

It ought to be apparent that just as an abnormal supply of unsaturated fatty acids requires additional vitamin E to prevent their peroxidation, so an abnormally large supply of oxygen would set up the same requirement. Nevertheless such a conclusion is better demonstrated than theorized about, and the Duke University research team set about performing an objective study with mice. They were able to demonstrate that vitamin E-deficient mice in a hyperbaric oxygen unit did develop hemolytic anemia and convulsions, whereas those whose diets were supplemented with vitamin E did not.

In conclusion the authors pointed out that their studies suggested that "certain manifestations of oxygen toxicity can be avoided in humans exposed to hyperoxia by pretreatment with vitamin E."

Thus vitamin E should not have been exactly unknown

to those planning the diets of astronauts. A year after the report of the Duke University study, it was reviewed in *Clinical Pharmacology and Therapeutics* (6: 6, pages 777-778) by Captain Carlos J. G. Perry of the U. S. Air Force Medical Corps. Captain Perry pointed out that, in addition to protection against peroxidation, vitamin E also has protective properties against extremes of temperature, hypoxia, and radiation exposure.

Yet in December of that same year, 1965, when Gemini 7 took off, the diet of the astronauts was supplemented with one gram of calcium a day to help counteract bone demineralization, but there was no vitamin E to protect them against the reductions in red cell mass and in blood plasma that had already been found after the Gemini 4 mission of McDivitt and White and the Gemini 5 mission of Cooper and Conrad.

It should have been known that the problem was bound to recur. Studies at the U. S. Army Medical Research and Nutrition Laboratory in Denver, Colorado, have shown very well that under conditions of high stress, it is not necessary for the diet to be high in polyunsaturates for the level of free fatty acids in the bloodstream to rise. They are mobilized from the triglyceride pool of adipose tissue. Their peroxidation in a pure oxygen atmosphere represented an obvious hazard, the answer to which was known but apparently ignored until 1969.

According to stories that appeared in the Toronto newspapers, the crew that circled the moon at Christmas 1968, again commanded by Colonel Borman, returned to earth showing a loss of between 20 and 30 per cent of their red blood cell mass. And so it was finally decided in preparing for the moon walk flight of Armstrong, Aldrin, and Collins, to supplement their diets with vitamin E as well as with calcium. In fact, they were given a full range of vitamins, since it was theorized that the dehydrated diet given them to save weight might be responsible for multiple vitamin deficiencies. In fact, the stripping of vitamin E from the diet during food processing is so universal that nearly everyone suffers from a vitamin E deficiency regardless of whether or not his food is dehydrated. If not, I have shown in the introductory chapter, there would probably be no coronary thrombosis.

In any case, we can probably be sure that the astronauts of the future will be well supplied with vitamin E on their voyages, and as a result, not only will they be spared the hemolytic anemia that has afflicted earlier crews, but they will also avoid the general weakening of the cardiovascular system that has been such a puzzle to the Aeronautics and Space Administration doctors.

CHAPTER 21. *ESTROGEN and ANTAGONISTS*

AS EXPLAINED IN CHAPTER I, THE whole concept underlying this work derived from the many pathological conditions that accompany hyperestrogenism and their correction by reducing the estrogen level to normal. At first, it was menorrhagia and dysmenorrhea that were successfully treated by my father and older brother and later by myself and younger brother. Then it was found that the alpha fraction of vitamin E could control the antiproteolytic factor found in the serum of aborting women and that it could prevent *abruptia placentae*, this between the years 1935 and 1937.

Gradually, it became apparent that there were at least four estrogen antagonists, namely progesterone, thyroid extract, alpha tocopherol, and testosterone and that these could be used singly or in combination. The result was a simple and effective method of treating the many conditions associated with the overproduction of estrogen by the body.

Most of these concepts have now been accepted. Paul Starr (116) for example, states without the need for reference that "in women during the reproductive years, hypothyroidism should be considered in any case of amenorrhea, infertility, habitual abortion, menorrhagia, or other menstrual disorders. It must be remembered that some of these cases are characterized by hyperestrogenism. . . ." No references are really necessary since most of the information was published between 1935 and 1942 over Dr. Evan Shute's name.

Since menorrhagia and dysmenorrhea respond so well to thyroid extract, that is if there is no other cause, such as fibroids or polyps or pelvic inflammatory disease, it follows that such patients must be hypothyroid. However, there really has been no accurate measure of low thyroid activity available until the advent of the Protein Bound Iodine and Iodine Uptake Tests. When these tests did become available, random samplings of the American population, especially one in the Chicago area, confirmed our long-standing and often-stated impression that there was a great deal of subclinical hypothyroidism. The Chicago study produced the figure of 55 per cent of females and 45 per cent of males in this category.

Before the days of the P.B.I. and the Iodine Uptake Test we relied entirely on a careful history and the physical examination of the patient. We long ago abandoned the Basal Metabolic Rate Test as inaccurate and misleading, in fact, useless. In this view, we have not been alone. Hamolsky and Freedberg (115) point out that the B.M.R. has been largely abandoned in many clinics and is being replaced by a therapeutic trial.

The patient with subacute hypothyroidism will have some but not necessarily all of the following symptoms: dry hair; dry skin, which if dry enough will often crack around the ends of the fingers or around the nails in winter; a tendency to gain weight easily, to have cold feet in bed (a very typical symptom), and to have one other symptom hard to describe in a few words. Many subclinical hypothyroids are slow starters, find it hard to get going in the morning, are usually doing at 11 o'clock what they ought to have done by nine o'clock and doing at four p.m. what they ought to have done by two p.m. However, as the day goes on they become more efficient, and by nine o'clock at night have "caught up" and are now full of life and ambition. They may be hard to get to bed at night and just as hard to get up in the morning. A woman who regularly irons at nine o'clock at night and sings as she irons, is a hypothyroid.

This symptom has nothing to do with intelligence or ambition. In fact, an overly energetic, highly educated young woman who became my patient was far from fat, served on several Y.W.C.A. boards, was engaged in several civic activities, played badminton and bridge, and was obviously a typical hyperthyroid until her history was taken in detail, when she became just as obviously a hypothyroid.

If the patient is a woman in her reproductive years, the diagnosis is much easier. She may have the typical symptoms associated with her menstrual cycle, the symptoms of overproduction of estrogen, namely, premenstrually sore, tender, and swollen breasts with a gain of weight due to water retention, irritability, and a heavy sensation in her abdomen. Her periods will usually be heavy, with clots, accompanied by dysmenorrhea and unduly prolonged. She may have pelvic pain at the time of ovulation.

On examination, she may obviously have the typical dry hair and skin, a poor outer third of the eyebrows, sideburns, beard, and mustache, and quite frequently hairs around the areola or between her breasts. Occasionally there will be a typical masculine distribution of pelvic hair with hair growing upwards to or toward the umbilicus. She is apt to have hairy legs.

These signs and symptoms are much more dependable than most tests. They make the diagnosis fairly certain, although a slow pulse is a necessary accompaniment, and in some forms of heart disease the pulse may not be slow until the heart condition comes under control.

It has become very obvious that the majority of cardiac and peripheral vascular disease patients that I see daily, are frankly hypothyroid and this condition must be corrected if possible, if complete treatment is to be attained.

Support for all this appeared unexpectedly and vividly when I came upon the feature article in *World Wide Abstracts of General Medicine*, (Vol. 5, no. 9, October, 1962) entitled "Subclinical Hypothyroidism — to treat or not to treat?" by Paul Starr (116). In it he states . . . "Chronic hypothyroidism results in the following disorders:

"1. Arteriosclerosis — especially of the brain.
"2. Myocarditis — sufficient to produce heart failure.
"3. Slow mentation, delayed comprehension, poor memory, loss of initiative.

"4. Atherosclerosis of the coronary arteries, with resulting angina pectoris.

"5. Anemia, resembling either the primary or secondary form.

"6. Somatic muscle weakness, leading to orthopedic disability.

"7. Anorexia and constipation, even to the point of obstruction.

"8. Fibrositis, with body-wide pains resembling gout.

"9. Phlebothrombosis, with resulting embolism."

Subsequently, he emphasizes the point, that "the citizen being damaged by hypothyroidism does not know it." In other words, it requires careful history taking and a knowledge of the physical signs and peculiar symptomatology to establish the diagnosis.

The patient correctly treated may well feel like a normal human being for the first time in his or her life, and the effect on the family that comes with the discovery of a different and more happy and efficient housewife is also a joy and a wonder.

One can always safely give the patient a clinical trial, starting at a safe level of crude or not too refined thyroid product and increasing until the desired effect is achieved, remembering that one out of ten who need thyroid can't take it, but that an overdosage is easy to detect and completely harmless as long as the drug is discontinued or reduced relatively promptly.

The hypothyroid female produces too much estrogen. This can nearly always be controlled by thyroid medication. If not detected and controlled she may well in later life develop the cardiovascular and other damage enumerated by Paul Starr and then need the full treatment with alpha tocopherol and thyroid.

CHAPTER 22. *HOPEFUL HORIZONS*

THERE ARE A FEW OTHER CONDItions in human medicine that we have treated successfully with alpha tocopherol, but in so few cases that it is not possible to state categorically what can be expected in a large series. For example, we have treated two cases of fragilitas ossium (a brittle condition of the bones), with conspicuous success, and have noted in the literature a report by Dr. Compere of Chicago, an orthopedic surgeon, on the successful treatment of a case of myositis ossificans, bony deposits and inflammation in muscle tissue.

I have treated two graduate nurses, who, following radical mastoidectomies, had persistent drainage from the ears of 20 and 25 years' duration, one with complete cure, the other with some help. We have treated with complete success several draining sinuses in osteomyelitis cases, one which was the result of a war wound. Unfortunately, the others were Workmen's Compensation Board cases, and they were immediately removed from our care by the board, as soon as our participation was learned. These patients were subjected to emergency radical surgery.

Therefore, the treatment of many and various types of cases must remain happy horizons!

Some rare conditions, how many no one can say until alpha tocopherol treatment is tried, respond to alpha tocopherol and to nothing else. Such a condition is epidermolysis bullosa dystrophica, an especially unpleasant skin disease.

The uses of alpha tocopherol in the obstetrical and

gynecological fields is certainly well established and widely confirmed, but, of course, not within the scope of this book. Note please that all this is due to the investigation of and the published work of my brother, Dr. Evan Shute.

Certainly our work has inspired a vast interest in the substance throughout the civilized world. Confirmations of the earliest work done are even now for the first time appearing in the medical literature.

Then, too, it is a matter of personal satisfaction that we were responsible for the excellent physical health of the astronauts as explained by Dr. David Turner on Canadian television. He is a biochemistry research associate at the Hospital for Sick Children in Toronto, Canada, and a consultant to the United States Aeronautics and Space Administration for both the Gemini and Apollo programs. When the astronauts who circled the moon last Christmas eve were examined, it was found that they had lost between 20 and 30 per cent of their red blood cell mass and that this loss of hemoglobin caused severe fatigue. Because Dr. Turner was in London, Canada, when we reported our work on vitamin E, the thought occurred to him that a deficiency in this vitamin might explain the astronauts' problem, and it proved to be so. This explanation and the solution were explored and published under N.A.S.A. sponsorship by Kann and associates in 1964, but apparently their work had been forgotten. So, once again, our work provided the solution to a most important problem, this time in space flight. Unfortunately, the astronauts and the members of their vast team will never know this, probably.

A most interesting comment of Dr. Turner's was his remark that the effect of vitamin E supplementation on the astronauts might lead to a breakthrough in the treatment of cardiac and other ailments!

The two previously mentioned cases of chronic suppuration and drainage continuing for years following mastoidectomy are interesting for two reasons. They were both nurses in the same Ontario Provincial Hospital, both had the same very common name, and both had mastoidectomies done over 20 years previously. Although working in the same hospital, they had never met; but the results achieved with treatment of the first case filtered through the hospital grapevine to the second one. Results with the first case, using alpha tocopherol by mouth, 600 units a day, was a complete disappearance of all discharge within four weeks, and it did not recur when there were subsequent head colds. The second case reported a diminution but not a disappearance of discharge, and it did not increase with subsequent head colds.

Theoretically, the reason for the continuing discharge in both parties was incomplete removal of infected bone cells and subsequent inadequate drainage. The first case may well have had adequate drainage; and with the increased blood supply in the bone cells immediately below the infected ones, they were able to slough off the diseased cells, just as happens routinely in our peripheral gangrenes. The second case may have differed in several ways, with more and deeper involvement of mastoid cells in the infective process, or may have had inadequate drainage and so have kept the cavity bathed in pus. Or, of course, this patient's lack of a more complete response to therapy could be due to an insufficient decrease in oxygen need.

The case of epidermolysis bullosa dystrophica was reported in detail in the *Canadian Medical Association Journal*, 90: 1315-1316, June 6, 1964. Reference is made in this article to three individual cases treated by their dermatologists with similar improvement.

Fragilitas Ossium —
Two Brief Case Reports

This rare disease, in which the bones are unusually fragile but in which fractures heal rapidly, has no ascertained cause and there has been no effective treatment. In many cases the usual treatment for any fracture that develops cannot be applied because either the apparatus used or the force necessary to accomplish reduction may cause fresh breaks. After a number of years the result can be numerous fractures with good healing but with poor alignment and, therefore, multiple deformities.

It may be interesting to report here two cases in which there has been apparent relief of the condition. Neither showed any evidences of rickets or syphilis.

Case 1. A blonde, blue-eyed baby girl with perhaps faintly blue sclera. The patient was the third child and was delivered uneventfully at term after a normal pregnancy. Her birth weight was six lbs. three oz. When the baby was brought home from the hospital, the parents noted that she did not use the left lower extremity. Her mother thought exercise was needed and provided it. The femur broke in her hands. Then an X-ray revealed a healing fracture of the hip as well as the fresh fracture of the femur. A month later, while dressing the baby, the mother lifted the baby's left hand and fractured the wrist. The following week the left tibia was fractured by trivial trauma.

When a month old the baby was given a series of injections of ACTH twice a week for six weeks, with no result, the two last fractures occurring during treatment. She has been treated from the age of four months with 200 I.U. of alpha tocopherol daily, as well as the usual amounts of calcium and vitamin D. There have been no fractures during the course of treatment, which is now of 11 months' duration.

Since the institution of alpha tocopherol treatment, the child has learned to crawl and stand up. She has fallen from her high-chair and from a sofa without injury.

Case 2. The second patient was discovered quite by accident. Her father, a cardiac patient treated for several months at the Shute Institute, developed pain in the chest and was put to bed in his daughter's bedroom. I called on him there and asked for a spoon to use as a tongue-depressor. I noticed they gave me a tongue-depressor from the dresser drawer, where they were kept together with every possible first aid item the daughter could require. My questions led to the information that this girl had been diagnosed as a case of fragilitas ossium and had learned to splint broken fingers and such minor fractures herself!

She is red-headed and aged 22. Her sclera are not bluish. She has been under alpha tocopherol treatment for over four months so far. However, in that time, she has twice fallen downstairs — once down a steel staircase in the university library and once at her home. She has had several other minor mishaps, which resulted in bruises and abrasions, but no fractures. She observes that these falls formerly would have led to fractures. Since preparing this report, she reports falling forward over the handle bars of a bicycle without fractures!

During the last five years she has had many fractures on small pretext. For example, she stumbled one time while going through a doorway; put her hand up to catch herself and broke two fingers. On another occasion, she put her foot in a stirrup to mount a horse and broke her ankle. In addition she has broken the bones of her left forearm and her nose after trivial trauma.

Her treatment in our hands has consisted of 300 I.U. of alpha tocopherol daily, as well as calcium and vitamin D.

We should point out that the mechanisms by which alpha tocopherol acts have been well-established by both animal and clinical investigation, and that it can be especially effective whenever there is a deficiency in tissue oxygenation or in blood supply. We theorized that alpha tocopherol could be tried in these two cases because it is a safe drug under these conditions; there is no other treatment; and theoretically there are tenuous reasons for associating it with calcium metabolism. It seems to have been effective.

An extension of the successful use of alpha tocopherol in treating kraurosis vulvae and leucoplakia vulvae with microscopically proven tissue rejuvenation reported by Dr. Evan Shute (117) led to its use in treating the one patient with leucoplakia of the vocal cords who ever applied to us for treatment.

This man, aged 47, was first seen on December 6, 1948 with involvement of both vocal cords. In June, 1947, a small nodule had been removed from the left cord, and the condition of leucoplakia was diagnosed at this time. Hoarseness recurred in November, 1947.

He was given 300 units of alpha tocopherol daily. He was due for a check-up on December 26, 1948 — three weeks after treatment began — and he was instructed to say nothing about the vitamin E treatment. This was important in his case since the otolaryngologist who was caring for him was attached to a major Detroit hospital, and his unbiased opinion was, therefore, very valuable.

As reported by the patient, the doctor said that "he had never seen such improvement." The same doctor made the same comment a month later and told the patient he need not report again for six months.

In June, 1949, the vocal cords were declared normal, and it was said that no one would suspect the diagnosis who had not seen the original condition.

Again, perhaps it was too small a series from which conclusions might be drawn, but at least this is one more hopeful horizon.

CHAPTER 23. *WHAT OF THE FUTURE?*

WHILE WORKING ON THIS BOOK, I have been asked many times what I really want from it. I hope it will be the means of making available to all sufferers from heart disease the help they deserve — a proven, successful treatment, so superior to any presently available that it makes the knowledgeable wonder whatever is the matter with organized medicine.

By now, most cardiologists must know they have nothing to offer but diagnosis and vague theories of the causation of a plague which threatens to engulf us as no plague or world war has ever been able to do. Many of these *must* know that there is a proven answer to the problem of clots. Certainly all surgeons must know of Dr. Alton Ochsner's work. How can it possibly be ignored much longer?

I hope the screams of the many victims of burns may be stilled and that they will avoid long and painful surgical treatments and grafts, that they will not end up with hideous scars and contraction deformities.

I hope that many gangrenous legs of diabetics may be saved, just as we have been saving them for years when no one else could.

I hope that many more men with poor blood supply to their legs may step out briskly again.

I do think that what is good enough for the astronauts is good enough for the American citizen, whose taxes pay for their training, and the many thousands of workmen and scientists who are involved in each flight. If they can get vitamin E, why can't everyone?

I hope that somehow the publicity-seeking heart transplant surgeons may cease to be heroes, since any medical man with such a record of failures would be read out of the profession.

Certainly many hundreds of patients with just as serious heart damage as most of the transplant victims have had years of comfortable life after receiving adequate treatment with alpha tocopherol, especially now that adequate diuretics are available.

I have lived long enough to see new medical discoveries change the whole course of serious disease. Insulin was discovered in Canada while I was an undergraduate, and it has meant years of health and life to millions.

While I was an interne in internal medicine in Chicago, a Dr. Robertson was brought all the way from the famous medical school in Peking, China, to work at the University of Chicago doing research in lobar pneumonia, in which he had already done some distinguished research work. As an interne, I took numerous nasal swabs, cultured sputum, and took material directly from the lungs, if necessary, to type the pneumococcus responsible for that particular patient's pneumonia. The patient was on a special bed with the mattress cut away behind his chest so that X-rays could be taken without disturbing him. In spite of some serum for specific strains, the mortality approximated 33 per cent, and the ones who survived often suffered with purulent pleural effusions and other complications. All were gravely ill for ten to 16 days. I had lost a beloved uncle and very nearly lost both my brothers with this disease. Then, along came the sulfonamides and the antibiotics. Lobar pneumonia and many acute and frequently fatal infections are now treated successfully and casually with a few pills and "call me if you're not better in a couple of days."

My father knew typhoid fever epidemic in spring and fall and saw many cases of diphtheria. I have made the diagnosis of typhoid fever once and have seen no cases of diphtheria.

My father saw few cases of coronary occlusion and few diabetics. I have seen thousands. There was *no* coronary thrombosis in 1900. There need be none in the year 1980. It's up to you now.

BIBLIOGRAPHY

(1) Dock, G. *Journ. Am. Med. Ass'n* 213: 583, 1939.
(2) Herrick, J. B., *Journ. Am. Med. Ass'n* 59: 2015, 1912.
(3) White, P. *Heart Disease,* Macmillan Co., New York, 1943.
(4) Malhotra, G. L. (India) *Brit. Heart J.* 29: 895, 1967.
(5) Morris, J. N. *Lancet* 1: landl: 69, 1951.
(6) Evans, H. M., Bishop, K. S. *J. Metab. Res.* 3: 233, 1923.
(7) Sure, B. *J. Biol. Chem.* 74: 45-53, July, 1927.
(8) Karrer, P., Escher, R., Fritsche, H., Keller, H., Ringier, B. H., and Salomon, H. *Helv. Chim. Acta* 21: 939, 1938.
(9) Zierler, K. L, Grob, D. and Lilienthal, J. L. (U.S.) *Am. J. Physiology* 153: 127, 1948.
(10) Houchin, O. B. and Mattill, H. A. (U.S.) *Proc. Soc. Exp. Biol. and Med.* 50: 216, 1942.
(11) Zierler, K. L., Folk, B. P., Eyzaguirre, C., Jarcho, L. W., Grob, D., and Lilienthal, J. L., *Ann. N.Y. Acad. Sci.* 52: 180, 1949.
(12) Levine, S. A. *Am. Heart J.* 42: 406, 1951.
also Levine, S. A. and Lown, B., *Journ. Am. Med. Ass'n.* 148: 1365, 1952.
(13) Goria, A. (Italy) *Boll. della Soc. Ital. di Biol. Sper.* 29: 1277, 1953.
(14) Goria, A. and Mallen, J. (Italy) *Boll. della Soc. Ital, di Biol. Sper.* 29: 1278, 1953.
(15) Leone, A. and Sulis, E. (Italy) *Ann. Ital. di Pediat.* Vol. 6: 1, 1953.
(16) Pult, H. (Germany) *Deutsche Med. Woch.* 79: 471, 1954.
(17) O'Connor, V. R. and Hodges, J. P. S. (England) International Congress on Vitamin E, Venice, Italy, Sept. 1955, P. 454.
(18) Puente-Dominguez, J. L. and Dominguez, R. *Rev. Espanola de Cardiologia* 9: 30, 1955.
(19) Lambert, N. H. (Eire) Proc. of Third Internat. Congress on Vitamin E, Venice, Italy, Sept. 1955.

(20) Ardissone, G. (Italy) *Rass. Internat. Clinica Ter.* 35: 345, 1955.

(21) Diaz, F. V. (Spain) *Progresos de Patol, y Clin.* 3: 351, 1956.

(22) Stepp, W. (W. Germany) *Med. Klin.* 53: 36, 1958.

(23) Shute, E. V. *J. Ob. and Gyn. Br. Emp.* 49: 482, 1942.

(24) Tusini, G. (Italy) *Boll. Soc. Lomb. Sci. Med. Biol.*, Mar. 15, 1949.

(25) Enria, G. and Ferrero, R. (Italy) *Arch. per la Scienze Mediche,* 91: 23, 1951.

(26) Edgerton, M. T., Hanrahan, E. M. and Davis, W. B. (U.S.) *Plastic and Reconstructive Surgery* 8: 224, 1951.

(27) Dominguez, J. P. and Dominguez, R. (Spain) *Angiologia* 5: 51, 1953.

(28) Calvi Lampetti, A. (Italy) Proc. Third Internat. Congress on Vitamin E, Venice, Italy, September, 1955, p. 453.

(29) Skelton, F., Shute, E. V., Skinner, H. G. and Waud, R.A. *Science* 103: 762, 1946.

(30) Fanfak, H. (Germany) *Aerztl. Forsch.* 6: 247, 1952.

(31) Shute, E. V., Vogelsang, A., Skelton, F. R. and Shute, W. E. *Surg. Gyn. and Obst.* 86: 1. 1948.

(32) Burgess, J. F. and Pritchard, J. E. (Canada) *Can M.A.J.* 59: 242, 1948.

(33) Dowd, G. C. (U.S.) *Annals N.Y. Acad. of Sciences* 52: 365, 1949.

(34) Stritzler, C. (U.S.) *Ann. N.Y. Acad. Sci.* 52: 368, 1949.

(35) Siedentopf, H. and Kruger, A. (Germany) *Sonder, Med. Klin.* 44: 1060, 1949.

(36) Anson, P. J. (Germany) *Landarzt* 26: 262, 1950.

(37) Block, M. T. (U.S.) *Clin. Medicine* 47: 112, 1950.

(38) Owings, J. C. (U.S.) See discussion of Ochsner, A., Kay, J. H., DeCamp, P. T., Hutton, S. B. and Balla, G. A. *Annals Surgery* 131: 652, 1950.

(39) Hagerman, G. (Sweden) *Archiv. f Dermat. u Syphillis,* 191: 637, 1950.

(40) Bierzynski, A. (West Indies) *Caribbean M. J.* 12: 5, 1950.

(41) Kemmer, C. H. (Poland) *Derm. Woch.* 126: 1209, 1952.

(42) Block, M. T. (U.S.) *Clin. Med.* 60: 1, 1953.

(43) Sidi, E. and Hincky, M. (France) *Gaz. Med. France* 60: 1361, 1953.

(44) Dalle Coste, P. and Klinger, R. (Italy) *Riforma Med.* 69: 853, 1955.

★(69) Reifferscheid, M. and Matis, P. (Germany) *Med. Welt.* 20: 1168, 1951.

(45) Lambert, N. H. (Eire) *Proc. Third International Congress on Vitamin E*, Venice, Italy, September, 1955, p. 610.

(46) Telford, I. R., Wiswell, O. B. and Smith, E. L. (U.S.) *Proc. Soc. Exp. Biol. and Med.* 87: 162, 1954.

(47) Telford, I. R., Wiswell, O. B., Smith, E. L., Clark, R. T., Jr., Tomashefski, J. F. and Criscuolo, D. (U.S.) Air University School of Aviation Medicine, Project No. 21-1201, 0013, Report, No. 4, May 1954 (Randolph Field, Texas).

(48) Saha, H. (India) *J. Indian Med. Assoc.* 23: 428, 1954.

(49) Molotchick, M. B. (U.S.) *Med. Record* 160: 667, 1947.

(50) Doumer, E., Merlen, J. and Dubruille, P. (France) *Presse Med.* 29: 394, 1949.

(51) Butturini, U. (Italy) *Gior di Clin. Med.* 31: 1, 1950.

(52) Dietrich, H. W. (U.S.) *South M. J.* 43: 743, 1950.

(53) Edgerton, M. T., Hanrahan, E. M. and Davis, W. B. (U.S.) *Plastic and Reconstructive Surgery* 8: 224, 1951.

(54) George, N. (Canada) *Summary* 3: 74, 1951.

(55) Terzani, G. (Italy) *Policlinica-Sezione Prat.* 58: 1381, 1951.

(56) Mosetti, A. and Boesi, S. (Italy) *Med. Internazionale* 60: 210, 1952.

(57) Romeo, F. and Parrinello, A. (Italy) *Acta Vitaminol.* 8: 129, 1954.

(58) Lee, P. F. (U.S.) *Summary* 8: 85, 1956.

(59) Keleman, E. and Lajos, I. (Hungary) *Orvosok Lapja* 5: 1603, 1948.

(60) Leinwand, I. (U.S.) *N. Y. State J. Med.* 48: 1503, 1948.

(61) de Oliviera, D. (Brazil) Separata de O Hospital, July, 1949.

(62) Boyd, A. M., Ratcliffe, A. H., James, G. W. and Jepson, R. P. (England) *Lancet* 2: 132, 1949.

(63) Heinsen, H. A. and Scheffler, H. (Germany) *Med. Woch.* 46: 909, 1951.

(64) Livingstone, P.D. and Jones, C. (England) *Lancet*, 2: 602, 1958.

(65) Houchin, O. B. and Smith, H. W. (U.S.) *Am. J. Physiol.* 141: 242, 1944.

(66) Kay, J. H., Hutton, S. B., Weiss, G. N. and Ochsner, A. (U.S.) *Surgery* 28: 124, 1950.

(67) Ochsner, A., DeBakey, M. E. and DeCamp, P. T. *J. Am. Med. Assoc.* 144: 831, 4, 1950.

(68) Bauer, R. (U.S.) *Wien. Klin. Woch.* 31: 552, 1951.

(70) Crump, W. E. and Heiskell, E. F. (U.S.) *Texas State J. of Med.* 48: 11, 1952.

(71) Krieg, E. (Germany) Published by Urban and Schwarzenberg, Munich, 1952.

(72) Vitak, B. (Czechoslovakia) *Ceskoslovenska Gynaekologie* 19: 345, 1954.

(73) Suffel, P. (Canada) *Can. M.A.J.* 74: 715, 1956.

(74) Kawahara, H. (Japan) *Nagoya J. of Med. Sci.* 22: 341, 1960.

(75) Garcia, C. C. (Spain) *Med. Espanola* 25: 345, 1951.

(76) Paul, R. M., Lewis, J. A. and De Luca, H. A. (Canada) *Can. J. Biochem. and Physiol.* 32: 347, 1954.

(77) Baguena, B. (Spain) *Rev. Med. de Liege* 5: 622, 1950

(78) Sternberg, J. and Pascoe-Dawson, E. (Canada) *Can. M.A.J.* 80: 266, 1959.

(79) Holman, R. T. (U.S.) *Am. J. Clin. Nutrition* 8: 95, 1960.

(80) Kingsbury, K. J. and Ward, R. J. (England) Letter to *Brit. M.J.* 1: 1538, 1961.

(81) Shute, W. E. *Urol. and Cut. Rev.* 50: 679, 1946.

(82) Prosperi, P. (Italy) *Acad. Med. Fisica Florentina*, March 10, 1949.

(83) Kunstmann, H. (Germany) *Medizinische* 35: 1195, 1955.

(84) Wilson, H. (Canada) *Can. M.A.J.* 90: 1315, 1964.

(85) Rapte, D. (Germany) *Pharm. Praxis.* 3: 59, 1965.

(86) Desanctis, P. N. and Furey, C. A. (U.S.) *J. Urol.* 97: 114, 1967.

(87) Johuda, E. and Miyita, H. (Japan) *J. Clin. Ophthalmology,* 17: 797, 1963.

(88) Hanna, M. B. (Egypt) *Bull. Ophth. Soc. Egypt,* 58: 219, 1965.

(89) Matolay, G. (Hungary) *Summary* 15: 14, 1963.

(90) Wojewski, A. and Roessler, R. (Poland) *Pol. Med. Sci., and History,* July, 1965 Bull, p. 110.

(91) Gerloczy, F. and Bencze, G. (Hungary) *Ernahrungsforschung* 7: 295, 1962.

(92) Gerloczy, F., Lancos, F., and Szabo, J. (Hungary) *Acta. Paediat. Acad. Sci. Hung.* 7: 363, 1966.

(93) Ochsner, A. (U.S.) Letter, *New Eng. J. Med.* 271: 211, 1964.

(94) Weinstock, B. S. (U.S.) *J. Am. Podiat. Assoc.* 51: 563, 1961.

(95) Matolay, G. (Hungary) *Summary* 15: 14, 1963.

(96) Boyd, A. M. and Marks, J. *Angiology,* 14: 198, 1963.

(97) Oldham, J. B. (Scotland) *J. Roy. Coll. Edinburgh* 9: 179, 1964.

(98) Prokop, L. (Germany) *Sportarztl. Prax.* 1: 19, 1960.
(99) Kamimura, M., Takahashi, S. and Henmi, I. (Japan) *Sapporo Med.* 21: 71, 1962.
(100) Nayar, M. S. (India) *Indian J. Physiol. and Pharmacol.* 8. 49, 1964.
(101) Ambrosio, L. D. and Pugliese-Carratelli, M. (Italy) *Rifoma. Med.* 68: 342, 1954. See *Summary* 7: 121, 1955.
(102) Govier, W. M., Yanz, N. and Grelis, M. E. (U.S.) *J. Pharmacol. and Exp. Ther.* 88: 373, 1946.
(103) Ochsner, A. (U.S.) *Postgraduate Medicine,* 44: 91, 1968.
(104) Antlitz, A. M., Valle, N. G. and Kosai, M. F. (U.S.) *South M.J.* 61: 307, 1968.
(105) Call, D. L. and Sanchez, M. (U.S.) *J. Nut.* 93: supp. Part II, October, 1967.
(106) Hauch, J. T., (Canada) *Can. M.A.J.* 77: 125, 1957.
(107) Kojima, K., Okajima, T., and Suzuki, M. (Japan) *Folia Ophthalmol.* Japan, 16: 323, 1965.
(108) Gerloczy, F., Bencze, B., Kassai, S. and Barto, L. (Hungary) *Gyermekgyogyaszat* 12: 225, 1961.
(109) Yudkin, J. (England) *Postgrad. Med.* 44: 67, 1968.
(110) Williams, H. T. G., Clein, L. J., and MacBeth, R. A., *C.M.A.J.* 87: 538, 1962.
(111) Toone, W. M. *Angiology,* 18, No. 7, July, 1967.
(112) Sherry, S. (U.S.) *Annals of Int. Med.* 69: 415, 1968.
(113) Short, D. *Brit. Med. J.* 4: 673-5, Dec. 14, 1968.
(114) Gullickson, T. W. and Calverley, C. E. (U.S.) *Science* 104: 312, 1946.
(115) Hamolsky, M. W., Freedberg, A. S. *New Engl. J. Med.* 262: January 7; 14; 21; 1960.
(116) Starr, P. *World Wide Abstracts of General Medicine,* Vol. 5, No. 9, Oct., 1962.
(117) Shute, E. V. *J.A.M.A.* 110: 889, 1938.
(118) Molotchick, M. B. (U.S.) *Med. Rec.* 160: 667, 1947.
(119) Lambert, N. H. (Eire) *Vet. Rec.* 27: 355, 1947.
(120) Pin, L. (France) Thesis, M. Lavergne, Paris, 1947.
(121) Dedichen, J. (Norway) *Nord. Med.* 41: 324, 1949.
(122) Steinberg, Cl. (U.S.) *Annals N.Y. Acad. Sci.* 52: 380, 1949.
(123) O'Connor, V. R. (England) *Medical World* 72: 299, 1950.
(124) Pendl, F. (Germany) *Deut. Med. Wochenschr.* 75: 1405, 1950.
(125) Goria, A. (Italy) *Boll. della Soc. Ital. di Biol. Sper.* 29: 1275, 1953.

INDEX

Alpha tocopherol, 13-23
Alpha tocopherol antagonists, 18, 191-194
Alpha tocopherol dosage, 18, 175-185
Alpha tocopherol ointment, 48, 139, 141, 165-169, 171-174
Angina pectoris, 20, 43-59, 177-178
Antihypertensive drugs, 35, 92-95
Antioxidant properties of alpha tocopherol, 21, 45
Antithrombin properties of alpha tocopherol, 11, 13-14, 22, 26-27
Arterial thrombosis, 133-135
Arteriosclerosis, 108
Atherosclerosis, 10, 51, 144

Bed rest, 19-20, 27-28, 32
Bibliography, 203-207
Birth defects, 97-105
Blood pressure (high), 11, 34-35, 91-95
Blood vessel diseases, 107-115
Blue babies, 97-105
Buerger's Disease, 108-109
Burns, 23, 163-169

Cardiovascular treatments, 15-23
Congenital heart disease, 97-105
Coronary Arterial Thrombosis, 133-135
Coronary heart disease, 51, 177-178
Coronary occlusion, 25-49, 179-181
Coronary thrombosis, 7-13, 24-42

Diabetes, 143-150
Diagnostic techniques, 87-90
Digitalis, 34
Dosages of alpha tocopherol, 175-185

Electrocardiogram, 87-90
Embolism, 133-135
Estrogen, 18, 191
Exercise, 110-111

Fragilitas Ossium, 195, 197-200

Gangrene, 145-147
Glomerulonephritis, 91, 144, 151-161

Heart surgery, 72-73, 97
Hemolytic anemia, 187-188
Hypertension, 11, 34-35, 91-95
Hypoxia, 44
Hypothyroidism, 192

Indolent ulcer, 137-141
Intercostal neuralgia, 47
Intermittent claudication, 107-111
Ischemic heart disease, 51-59

Kidney disease, 151-161

Levine, Dr. Samuel, 27, 29-32

Mastoidectomies, 195
Myocardial infarction, 10, 31

Nitroglycerin, 45

Ochsner, Dr. Alton, 27, 33, 127-128
Oral contraceptives, 128
Oxygen toxicity, 187-188

Peripheral Vascular disease, 23 107-115, 145
Physical activity, 32
Polyunsaturated fats, 45, 80
Pulmonary embolism, 126-128
Purpura, 15

Rare diseases, 195-200
Reproductive disorders, 14
Retinal changes in diabetes, 147-149
Rheumatic fever, 61-69
Rheumatic heart disease (acute), 61-69, 181-182
Rheumatic heart disease (chronic), 71-86, 182-185

Saturated fats, 9
Skelton, Dr. Floyd, 15
Space medicine, 187-190, 196
Status Anginosis, 49
Stress, 8, 32
Surgical treatments, 72-74 97-100, 118-119

Thrombophlebitis, 125-135

Ulcers (leg), 137-141
Unsaturated fats, 188

Varicose veins, 117-124
Venous thrombosis, 27, 125-132
Vitamin E ointment, 48, 139-141